All About Nutrition

(Make your own Diet)

Diet preparation tools with basic understanding
(First Edition)

Authors:
Mr. Hitesh Andel
(Dietitian and wellness Coach)
Asst. Prof. Vandana Andel
M.Sc (Nursing)-**Community Health Nursing**
Mr. Ritesh Andel
B.Sc (Nursing) R&D in Wellness, **CHO**

DISCLAIMER

This book is solely written based on my personal experience and I, in no way claim that the information in it is 100% verified, as there are more and more researches coming every day, discretion is advised.
Furthermore, nothing contained herein is intended for the treatment or prevention of disease, nor as a substitute for medical treatment, nor as an alternative to medical advice.
Use of any supplements/drugs and exercise regimen should only be done under the directions and auspices of a licensed physician.
The writer does not claim to be a medical doctor nor does he purport to issue medical advice.
The guidelines herein are at the sole choice and risk of the reader.

For information contact:
Email: Fitnessndietitianadda@gmail.com
Instagram: fitnessndietitianadda
YouTube: Fitness & Dietitian Adda™

Index

INTRODUCTION

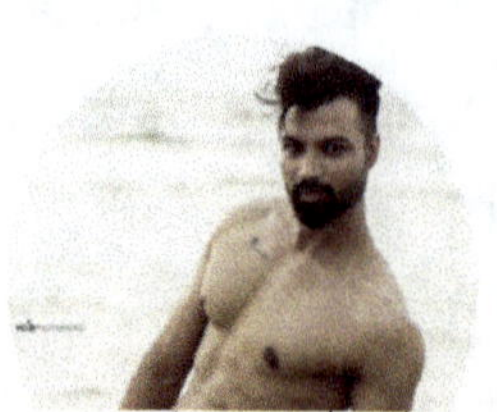

There are so many people who are conscious about health and fitness, but they don't find the right track to move forward. They're dependent on others to get fit. But sometimes it's confusing to hear anyone because many people give their opinion, and what is right for us, we never know.

So the solution is here, this book will try to teach you how to plan your own diet as per your need. I've tried to teach very basic things which are needed to prepare a diet.

As when I started my fitness career in 2009, I heard so many bodybuilders. Once upon a time I used to follow Youtubers but there was also some confusion as one is saying different things and the other one is different on the same topic.

But thereafter I started reading the experts and applying the things on me and when I started getting results I began to apply the research on my clients with some alteration as per their body needs.

All the facts I found during my research I've put all those topics in this book, because at that time those questions I was facing, not only mine but I've come to know that the same questions also have the maximum number of people.

I'm pretty much sure this book is going to help you a lot, whether you are beginner, intermediate or an advanced level athlete.

In 2019, I was preparing for Natural Bodybuilding Competition Federation "I Compete Natural" - ICN (Australia). When I was preparing for the competition I learned different things and applied myself and the result was positively awesome. That was the first competition of my life.

So be ready to learn the basic concepts of planning your own as well as your friends or family's diet too.

Author/-

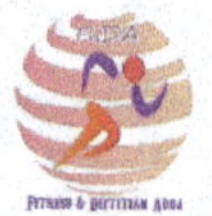

4

Chapter 1: Nutrition

Nutrition in Ancient India

In the pre-agricultural era, entire mankind consumed meat as early man was a hunter. Possibly he ate from plant sources which grew in the wilderness. With the advent of agriculture as an outcome of civilization, man acquired the ability to cultivate what he wanted, as by now he was influenced to some extent by the selection of the food that he wanted to eat.

All this ultimately led to him taking to vegetarianism, which probably did not occur until approximately 1500 B.C.

It is tried in this study to examine the concept of nutrition, balanced diet, appetite, food etiquette, food sanitation and food poisoning etc. in ancient India.

People in ancient India had an intuitive knowledge about nutrition, as proved by the 'Mahamrityunjaya mantra', which talks about sustenance when talking about the deity. People always knew their local produce and food options. More often than not, access to high-quality food was the problem.

However, that is not the only issue when it comes to nutrition as there is religious, philosophical and political bias as well. Traditional food in the country was vegan, organic and balanced in its own manner in different regions of ancient India.

For example, *Idli is served with sambar, and bajre ki roti is served with gud* and such balancing acts have always been part of Ayurvedic, Yunani and modern medicine culture.

Nutrition Theory

The concept of metabolism, the transfer of food and oxygen into heat and water in the body, creating energy, was discovered in 1770 by Antoine Lavoisier, the *"Father of Nutrition and Chemistry."*

Antoine Lavoisier (1743-94) showed that O_2 consumption increased during work, exposure to cold and during digestion (specific dynamic effect), and was lower during fasting (basal metabolism).

Meaning of word Nutrition

The word 'Nutrition' is derived from the late Latin word 'nutrire' which means to feed or to nourish.

Nutrition is very important to lead a healthy life. A balanced diet reduces the risk of diseases and improves the overall health of an

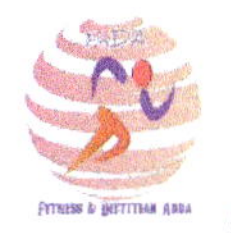

organism. It provides energy to the cells to carry out the cellular activities.

Human nutrition is the science of diet and its interactions with growth, development, physiology, metabolism, and composition of the human body. It involves the role of nutrition in normal and abnormal individuals, the impact of nutrition on health and disease, and the interactions between **diet, host, and environment**.

Definition of Nutrition

Nutrition is defined as,

"The processes by which an animal or plant takes in and utilises food substances."

Medical Definition of Nutrition

1. The process of taking in food and using it for growth, metabolism, and repair. Nutritional stages are ingestion, digestion, absorption, transport, assimilation, and excretion.
2. A nourishing substance, such as nutritional solutions delivered to hospitalized patients via an IV or IG tube.

Types of Nutrition

The mode of nutrition varies from one species to another. Broadly, there are two modes of nutrition among living organisms, namely:

1. **Autotrophic mode**
2. **Heterotrophic mode**

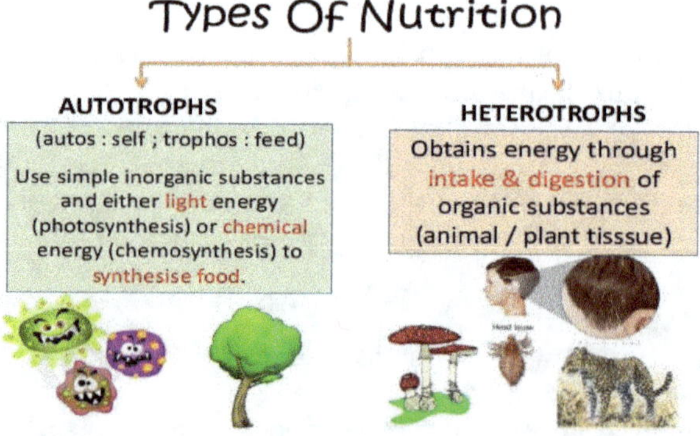

Autotrophic mode

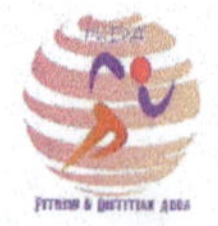

In the autotrophic mode, organisms use simple inorganic matters like water and carbon dioxide in the presence of light and chlorophyll to synthesize food on their own. In other words, the process of photosynthesis is used to convert light energy into food such as glucose. Such organisms are called autotrophs. Plants, algae, and bacteria (cyanobacteria) are some examples where autotrophic nutrition is observed.

During photosynthesis, carbon dioxide and water get converted into carbohydrates. These carbohydrates are stored in the form of starch in plants. Plants later derive the energy required from the stored starch. The process of photosynthesis can be explained in three stages:

1. **Absorption**: The chlorophyll present in leaves traps the light coming from the sun.
2. **Conversion**: The absorbed light energy gets converted into chemical energy. And water absorbed will split into hydrogen and oxygen molecules.
3. **Reduction**: At last, carbon dioxide gets reduced i.e. hydrogen molecules combine with carbon, to form carbohydrates (sugar molecules).

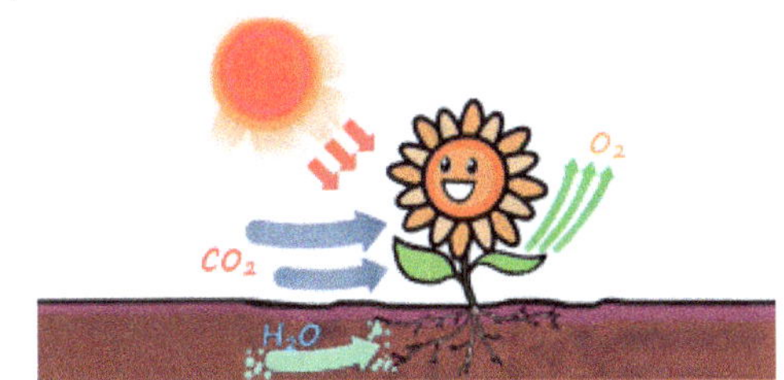

$$6CO_2 + 12H_2O \xrightarrow[\text{Chlorophyll}]{\text{Sunlight}} C_6H_{12}O_6 + 6O_2 + 6H_2O$$

All three events are not a continuous process. They may or may not take place sequentially.

In plants, stomata are the openings on leaves where gaseous exchange takes place and is regulated by guard cells. Plants take in and release gases through these stomatal pores.

In desert-like habitats, to avoid water loss, guard cells keep these pores closed during the daytime. Later, during the night time, stomata will be opened to absorb carbon dioxide and stored in the vacuoles. During the daytime, they will use this stored carbon dioxide

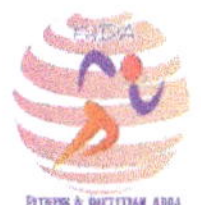

to perform *photosynthesis*. Other than *photosynthesis*, plants also depend on soil for micro and macro elements. These elements are used to synthesize proteins and other essential compounds required for the proper functioning and growth of the plants.

Heterotrophic mode

Every organism is not capable of preparing food on its own. Such organisms *depend on others* for their nutrition. The organisms which cannot produce food on their own and depend on Other sources/organisms are called heterotrophs. This mode of nutrition is known as heterotrophic nutrition.

Fungi and all the animals including humans are heterotrophs. Heterotrophs can be of many varieties depending upon their environment and adaptations. Some may eat plants (herbivores) and others eat animals (carnivores) while few eat both (omnivores). Thus we can say survival of heterotrophs depends directly or indirectly on plants.

Heterotrophs are classified into different categories based on their mode of nutrition. They are:

- Parasites (e.g. leeches, ticks)
- Saprophytes (e.g. mushrooms)
- Holozoic (e.g. humans, dogs)

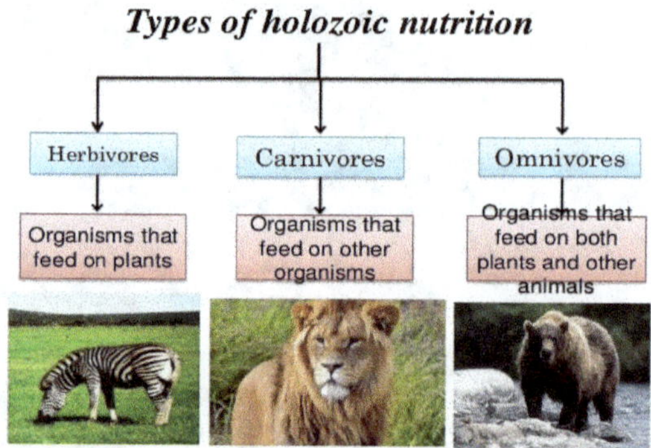

Importance / Need of Nutrition

Nutrition is very much essential for an organism. Best nutrition not only promotes better physical health and decreases sensitivity to disease, but also participates in cognitive development and academic achievement. *Nutrition promotes growth and development*. It keeps an organism healthy and wellbeing. Nutrition *prevents future illness and improves the length and quality of life*. The body needs nutrition for proper functioning and metabolism.

- Nutrition is necessary for the growth of new cells and the replacement or repair of worn-out cells.
- Nutrition gives energy for different metabolic processes in the body.
- Nutrition is required to produce resistance against different diseases.
- The substrate for energy production which is utilized in the different life processes for survival is provided by nutrition.

_______________________By_Mr._Hitesh_Andel_______________________

Chapter 2: Nutrient

Meaning of Nutrient

Nutrients are the substances which provide energy and biomolecules necessary for carrying out the various body functions. All living organisms need nutrients for proper functioning and growth. But they show divergence in how they fulfill this demand. Some animals feed on simple inorganic compounds to meet their nutrient requirement, while others utilise complex compounds.

Nutrients are **compounds in foods essential to life and health**, providing us with energy, the building blocks for repair and growth and substances necessary to regulate chemical processes.

Essential nutrients include **protein, carbohydrate, fat, vitamins, minerals and electrolytes**. Normally, *85% of daily energy use is from fat and carbohydrates and 15% from protein.*

Types of Nutrients

1. Macronutrients
2. Micronutrient

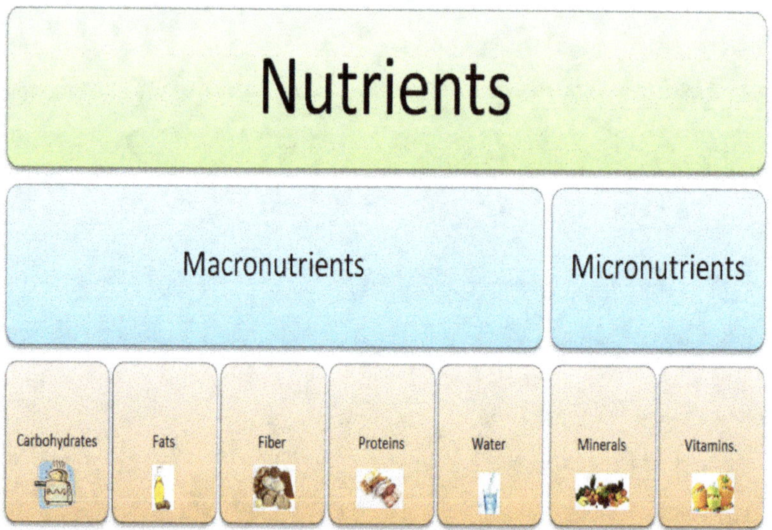

Macronutrients

Macronutrients are nutrients that provide calories or energy and are required in large amounts to maintain body functions and carry out the activities of daily life. There are three broad classes of macronutrients: proteins, carbohydrates and fats.

Micronutrients

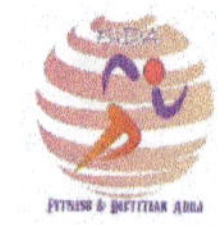

Micronutrients are one of the major groups of nutrients your body needs. They include vitamins and minerals. Vitamins are necessary for energy production, immune function, blood clotting and other functions. Meanwhile, minerals play an important role in growth, bone health, fluid balance and several other processes.

MICRONUTRIENTS	MACRONUTRIENTS
Micronutrients are required in small quantities	Macronutrients are required in large quantities.
They are present in low concentration in plant.	They are present in excessive concentration in plant.
They are also called trace elements	Also called as major elements
Examples: Fe, Mn, Cu, Zn, Mo, B, Cl, and Ni.	Examples: C, H, O, N,P, K, Ca, S, and Mg.
All micronutrients are minerals.	Majority of macronutrients are minerals, some are non-minerals (C, H and O).
They can be toxic for the plant if present excess in the cell than the required quantity.	They are usually not toxic to the cell if they are present in relatively higher concentration than the normal level.

They are collectively six major nutrients:

- Carbohydrates (CHO)
- Proteins,
- Lipids (fats),
- Vitamins,
- Minerals,
- Water.

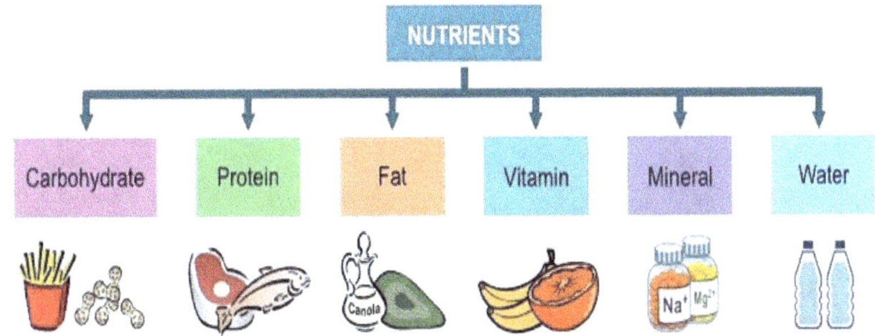

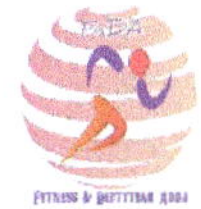

Functions of Nutrients

Carbohydrates
  energy and fiber source

Protein
  structural building blocks

Fat
  energy storage; cell repair

Water
  solvent and lubricant;
  transport of nutrients;
  temperature regulation

Vitamins
  involved in chemical reactions

Minerals
  involved in enzyme functions,
  nerve impulses, and bone structure

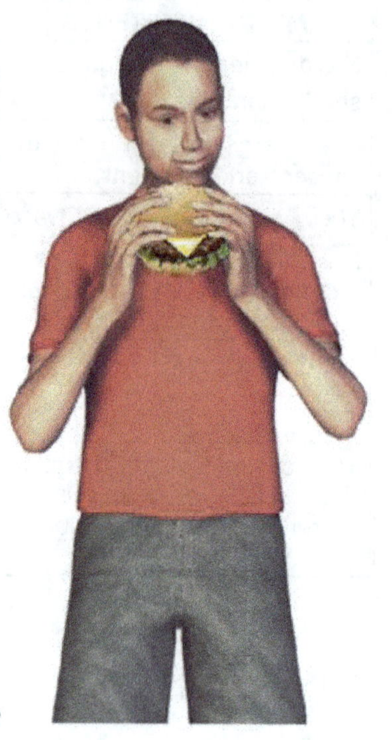

Carbohydrates (CHO)

Mainly sugars and starches, together constituting one of the three principal types of nutrients used as energy sources (calories) by the body. Carbohydrates can also be defined chemically as neutral compounds of carbon, hydrogen and oxygen.

Protein

Chemically, protein is composed of amino acids, which are organic compounds made of carbon, hydrogen, nitrogen, oxygen or sulfur. Your body needs protein to stay healthy and work the way it should. More than 10,000 types are found in everything from your organs to your muscles and tissues to your bones, skin, and hair. Protein is also a critical part of the processes that fuel your energy and *carry oxygen throughout your body in your blood.*

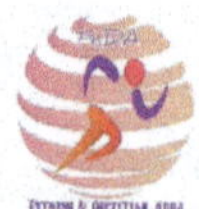

12

Lipids (Fats)

Lipids are fat-like substances found in your blood and body tissues. Your body needs small amounts of lipids to work normally.

Major types include fats and oils, waxes, phospholipids, and steroids. Fats are made up of fatty acids and either glycerol or sphingosine.

Lipids can be more formally defined as substances such as a fat, oil or wax that dissolves in alcohol but not in water. Lipids are easily stored in the body.

Vitamins

Vitamins are substances that our bodies need to develop and function normally. They include vitamins A, C, D, E, and K, choline, and the B vitamins (thiamin, riboflavin, niacin, pantothenic acid, biotin, vitamin B6, vitamin B12, and folate/folic acid).

Mineral

A mineral is a naturally occurring inorganic solid, with a definite chemical composition, and an ordered atomic arrangement. Minerals are substances that are formed naturally in the Earth. A mineral can be made of a single chemical element or more, usually a compound.

A mineral is a natural substance with distinctive chemical and physical properties, composition, and atomic structure.

Water

Water, a substance composed of the chemical elements hydrogen and oxygen and existing in gaseous, liquid, and solid states. It is one of the most plentiful and essential of compounds. A tasteless and odourless liquid at room temperature, it has the important ability to dissolve many other substances.

Importance of Nutrients

Nutrients are compounds in foods essential to life and health, providing us with energy, the building blocks for repair and growth and substances necessary to regulate chemical processes.

Nutrition Vs. Nutrient

Nutrients are substances that are required for the nourishment of organisms while *Nutrition* is the entire process by which organisms obtain energy and nutrients from food.

Carbohydrates, proteins, fats, vitamins and minerals are essential components of food, these components are called *Nutrients*, but

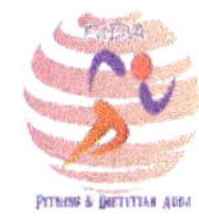

Nutrition is the mode of taking food by an organism and its utilisation by the body.

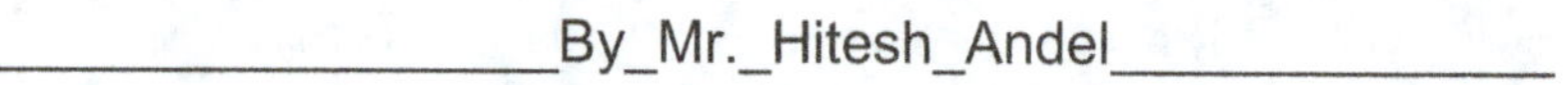

________________________By_Mr._Hitesh_Andel_______________

Chapter 3: Carbohydrates

Meaning

Carbohydrates, or carbs, are sugar molecules. Along with proteins and fats, carbohydrates are one of three main nutrients found in foods and drinks. Your body breaks down carbohydrates into glucose. *Glucose, or blood sugar, is the main source of energy for your body's cells, tissues, and organs.*

Carbohydrates are the body's main source of energy. In their absence, your body will use protein and fat for energy. It may also be hard to get enough fibre, which is important for long-term health.

Carbohydrates: Mainly sugars and starches, together constituting one of the three principal types of nutrients used as energy sources (calories) by the body. Carbohydrates can also be defined chemically as neutral compounds of carbon, hydrogen and oxygen(CHO).

Types of Carbohydrates

- Simple Carb
- Complex Carb

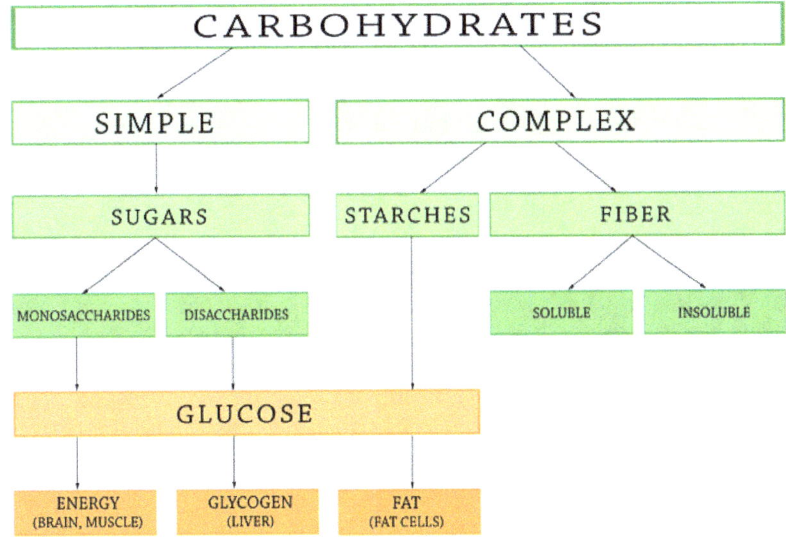

Simple carbohydrates:

These are also called *simple sugars.* Simple carbohydrates are broken down quickly by the body to be used as energy. Simple carbohydrates are found naturally in foods such as fruits,

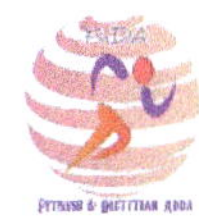

15

milk, and milk products. They are also found in processed and refined sugars such as candy, table sugar, syrups, and soft drinks. If you have a lollipop, you're eating simple carbs. But you'll also find simple sugars in more nutritious foods, such as fruit and milk. It's healthier to get your simple sugars from foods like these. Why? Because sugar isn't added to them and they also contain vitamins, fiber, and important nutrients like calcium. A lollipop has lots of added sugar and doesn't contain important nutrients.

Sugar: - Glucose, Fructose (a.k.a. fruit sugar), Sucrose (a.k.a. table sugar), Lactose (a.k.a. dairy sugar.
- ☐ ***Monosaccharides** are simple (unit) sugars.*
- ☐ ***Disaccharides** consist of molecules whose form is that of two monosaccharide molecules joined together.*

Complex carbohydrates:

These are also called *starches*. Starches include grain products, such as bread, crackers, pasta, and rice. As with simple sugars, some complex carbohydrate foods are better choices than others. **Refined grains, such as *white flour* and *white rice*, have been processed, which *removes nutrients and fiber*.** But unrefined grains **still contain these Vitamins and minerals**. They're also rich in fiber, which helps your digestive system work well.

Fiber helps you feel full, so you're less likely to overeat. *A bowl of oatmeal fills you up better than sugary candy with the same amount of calories.*

Starch : Starch is a carbohydrate commonly found in nature and one of the primary *sources of food energy* for human beings. It is *regularly eaten in the form of wheat, rice, potatoes, and other staple foods cultivated* throughout the world.

Fiber : Fibre is made up of the indigestible parts or compounds of plants, which pass relatively unchanged through our stomach and intestines. Fibre is mainly a carbohydrate. The main role of fibre is to keep the digestive system healthy.

There are 2 different types of Fiber :-
- ☐ Soluble
- ☐ Insoluble

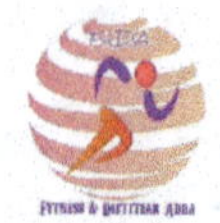

16

Soluble fiber attracts water and turns to gel during digestion. This slows digestion. Soluble fiber is found in oat bran, barley, nuts, seeds, beans, lentils, peas, and some fruits and vegetables. It is also found in psyllium *(ispaghula)*, a common fiber supplement. Some types of soluble fiber may help lower risk of heart disease.

Insoluble fiber is found in foods such as wheat bran, vegetables, and whole grains. It adds bulk to the stool and appears to help food pass more quickly through the stomach and intestines.

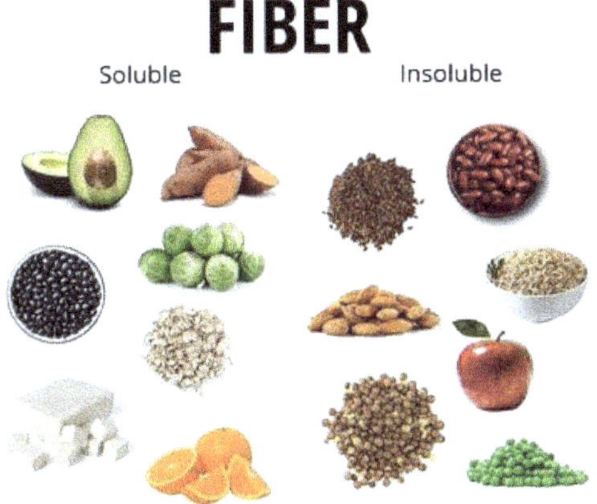

Some Important Points

"Glucose is the main source of fuel for our cells. When the body doesn't need to use the glucose for energy, it stores it in the liver and muscles. This stored form of glucose is made up of many connected glucose molecules and is called glycogen."

"Glycogen is stored in liver and muscle cells and is a secondary source of energy to freely circulating blood glucose. When the body needs more energy, certain proteins called enzymes break down glycogen into glucose. They send the glucose out into the body."

After a meal, carbohydrates are broken down into glucose, an immediate source of energy. Excess glucose gets stored in the liver as glycogen or, with the help of insulin, converted into fatty acids, circulated to other parts of the body and stored as fat in adipose tissue. When there is an overabundance of fatty acids, fat also builds up in the liver.

17

In simple words, **When your liver can not hold more glycogen, insulin triggers your fat cells to take-in glucose.**

Good vs. Bad Carbs

Good	Bad
non-starchy vegetables	soda
starchy vegetables	white pasta
fruits	white rice
greens	sugary cereal

Function: How Does the Body Use Carbs?

When you eat carbs, your body breaks them down into simple sugars, which are absorbed into the bloodstream. As the sugar level rises in your body, the pancreas releases a hormone called insulin.

Insulin is needed to move sugar from the blood into the cells, where the sugar can be used as an energy source.

When this process goes fast — as with simple sugars — you're more likely to feel hungry again soon.

When it goes more slowly, as with a whole-grain food, you'll be satisfied longer. These types of complex carbs give you energy over a longer period of time.

The carbs in some foods (mostly those with a lot of simple sugars) make the blood sugar level rise more quickly than others. Scientists have been studying whether eating foods that cause big jumps in blood sugar may be related to health problems like diabetes and heart disease.

You're probably already on the right track if you're limiting simple sugars (such as candy) and eating more complex carbs (like vegetables, oatmeal, and whole-grain wheat bread).

Carb Deficiency

When you don't get enough carbohydrates, the level of sugar in your blood may drop to below the normal range (70-99 mg/dL), causing hypoglycemia. Your body then starts to burn fat for energy, leading to ketosis.

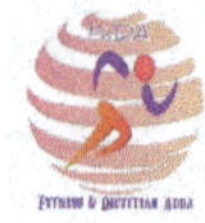

"Ketosis is a process that happens when your body doesn't have enough carbohydrates to burn for energy. Instead, it burns fat and makes things called ketones, which it can use for fuel."

Symptoms of hypoglycemia include:
- Hunger
- Shakiness
- Dizziness
- Confusion
- Difficulty speaking
- Feeling anxious or weak

Symptoms of ketosis include:
- Mental fatigue
- Bad breath
- Nausea and headache
- Painful swelling of the joints and kidney stones in severe ketosis

Carb Surplus

A diet too high in refined carbohydrates may cause sugar spikes and crashes dubbed "the blood sugar roller coaster," which increases the risk for Diabetes. Long-term high-carbohydrate diets with reduced fat and/or protein intake may lead to symptoms associated with essential fatty acid deficiency or essential amino acid deficiency.

These include:
- Dry skin
- Weak muscles
- Fatty food craving
- Depression

Source of Carbs

Carbohydrates are found in a wide array of both healthy and unhealthy foods—*bread, beans, milk, popcorn, potatoes, cookies, spaghetti, soft drinks, corn, and cherry pie.* They also come in a variety of forms. The most common and abundant forms are *sugars, fibers, and starches.*

Common foods with carbohydrates include

- **Grains**, (noodles, pasta, crackers, cereals, and rice)
- **Fruits**, (apples, bananas, berries, mangoes, melons, and oranges)
- **Dairy products**, (milk and yogurt)

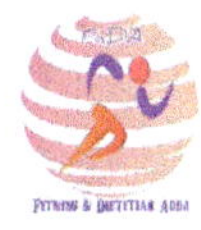

19

- **Legumes**, (dried beans, lentils, and peas)
- **Snack foods and sweets**, (cakes, cookies, candy, and other desserts)
- **Juices**, (regular sodas, fruit drinks, sports drinks, and energy drinks that contain sugar)
- **Starchy vegetables**, (potatoes, corn, and peas)

Some foods don't have a lot of carbohydrates, such as meat, fish, poultry, some types of cheese, nuts, and oils.

You do need to eat some carbohydrates to give your body energy. But it's important to eat the right kinds of carbohydrates for your health:

- **When eating grains, choose mostly whole grains and not refined grains:**
  - **Whole grains** are foods like whole wheat bread, brown rice, whole cornmeal, and oatmeal. They offer lots of nutrients that your body needs, like vitamins, minerals, and fiber. To figure out whether a product has a lot of whole grain, check the ingredients list on the package and see if a whole grain is one of the first few items listed.
  - **Refined grains** are foods that have had some of the grains removed. This also removes some of the nutrients that are good for your health.
- **Eat foods with lots of fiber.** The Nutrition Facts label on the back of food packages tells you how much fiber a product has.
- **Try to avoid foods that have a lot of added sugar.** These foods can have many calories but not much nutrition. Eating too much added sugar raises your blood sugar and can make you gain weight. You can tell if a food or drink has added sugars by looking at the Nutrition facts label on the back of the food package. It tells you how much total sugar and added sugar is in that food or drink.

How many carbohydrates should I eat?

There is no one-size-fits-all amount of carbohydrates that people should eat. This amount can vary, depending on factors such as your age, sex, health, and whether or not you are trying to lose or gain weight.

On average, people should get 45 to 65% of their calories from carbohydrates every day. On the Nutrition Facts labels, the Daily Value for total carbohydrates is 275 g per day. This is based on a

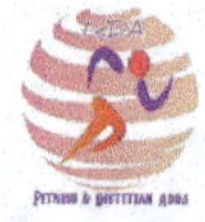

20

2,000-calorie daily diet. Your Daily Value may be higher or lower depending on your calorie needs and health.

Is it safe to eat a low-carb diet?

Some people go on a low-carb diet to try to lose weight. This usually means eating 25g and 150g of carbs each day. This kind of diet can be safe, but you should talk to your health care provider before starting it. One problem with low-carb diets is that they can limit the amount of fiber you get each day. They can also be hard to stay on for the long term.

Healthy Carbs and Complex Carbs List

Simple and complex carbohydrates can be misunderstood. Since whole fruit is a simple carb, it's best to categorize carbs as either bad or good carbs. Here's your complete good healthy carbohydrates list. (Carb grams for most packaged foods can be found on the label.)

NUTS & SEEDS	AMOUNT	CARBS*	WHOLE GRAINS	AMOUNT	CARBS*
Almonds	1 oz	6	Bread, whole wheat	1 slice	14
Brazil nuts	1 oz	4	Bread, multi grain	1 slice	17
Cashews	1 oz	9	Oatmeal, cooked	1 cup	25
Coconut, raw	1 oz	4	Pancake, buckwheat mix	1/3 cup (3 cakes)	33
Macadamia nuts	1 oz	4	Pancake, whole grain mix	1/3 cup (3 cakes)	28
Peanuts	1 oz	6	Pasta, whole wheat	1 cup cooked	37
Pecans	1 oz	5	Popcorn, popped	3-1/2 cups	19
Pistachios	1 oz	7	Rice, basmati brown	1/4 cup dry	31
Pumpkin seeds	1 oz	5	Rice, brown	1/4 cup dry	33

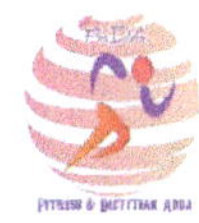

21

Sesame seeds	1 Tbsp	1	Rice, brown	1/2 cup cooked	22
Sunflower	1 oz	5	Rice, wild	1/2 cup cooked	18
Walnuts	1 oz	3	Rye bread	1 slice	15

BEANS & PEAS	AMOUNT	CARBS*	FRUITS (raw)	AMOUNT	CARBS*
Black beans	1/4 cup dry	23	Apple	5 oz	21
Black beans	1/2 cup cooked	18	Apricot	3 (4 oz ea.)	12
Chickpeas	1/4 cup dry	28	Avocado	1/2 (3 oz)	7
Chickpeas	1/2 cup cooked	18	Blackberries	1 cup	18
Kidney beans	1/4 cup dry	29	Blueberries	1 cup	21
Kidney beans	1/2 cup cooked	20	Cantaloupe	1 cup	13
Lentils	1/4 cup dry	28	Cranberries	1/2 cup	6
Lentils	1/2 cup cooked	20	Grapefruit	1/2 (4 oz)	10
Lima Beans	1/4 cup dry	22	Grapes	1 cup	16
Lima Beans	1/2 cup cooked	20	Guava	1 (3 oz)	11
Navy Beans	1/4 cup dry	32	Kiwi	1 (2-1/2 oz)	11
Navy Beans	1/2 cup cooked	29	Mango	1/2 (3-1/2 oz)	18
Pinto Beans	1/4 cup dry	29	Nectarine	1 (5 oz)	16
Pinto Beans	1/2 cup cooked	22	Orange	1 (4-1/2 oz)	15
Soybeans	1/4 cup dry	13	Papaya	1/2(5-1/2 oz)	15
Soybeans	1/2 cup cooked	9	Peach	1 (3-1/2 oz)	10
Split Peas	1/4 cup dry	26	Pier	1 (6 oz)	25
Split Peas	1/2 cup cooked	21	Pineapple	1 cup	19

	AMOUNT	CARBS*		AMOUNT	CARBS*
			Raspberries	1 cup	14
VEGETABLES	**AMOUNT**	**CARBS***	Strawberries	1 cup	11
Onions	1/2 cup cooked	7	Tangerine	1 (3 oz)	9
Radishes	1/2 cup raw	2	Watermelon	1 cup	12
Red Bell Peppers	1/2 cup raw	3			
Red Cabbage	1/2 cup cooked	4	VEGETABLES	AMOUNT	CARBS*
Romaine lettuce	1-1/2 cups raw	2	Alfalfa sprouts, raw	1/2 cup	1
Scallions	1/2 cup raw	4	Asparagus	1/2 cup cooked	4
Spinach	1/2 cup cooked	3	Butterhead lettuce	1 cup raw	2
Swiss Chard	1/2 cup cooked	4	Broccoli	1/2 cup cooked	4
Zucchini	1/2 cup cooked	4	Brussels Sprouts	1/2 cup cooked	7
			Cabbage	1/2 cup cooked	4
DAIRY	**AMOUNT**	**CARBS***	Carrot	1 (2-1/2 oz)	7
Blue cheese	1 oz	0.7	Cauliflower	3 florets	3
Cheddar cheese	1 oz	0.4	Celery	1/2 cup diced	2
Cottage cheese, 2% fat	1/2 cup	4	Chinese Cabbage	1/2 cup cooked	2
Egg	1 extra large	1	Chili Peppers	1 Tbsp	1
Feta cheese	1 oz	1	Corn (sweet)	1 ear	19
Milk, 1% fat	1 cup	8	Cucumber	5 oz raw	4
Milk, fat-free	1 cup	13	Edamame, fresh soybeans	1/2 cup raw	14
Mozzarella cheese	1 oz	0.8	Edamame	1/4 cup cooked	10
Parmesan cheese	1 Tbsp.	0.2	Eggplant	1/2 cup cooked	3

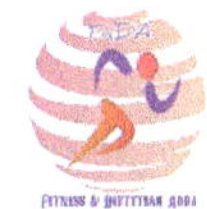

23

Provolone cheese	1 oz	0.6	Garlic	1 clove	1
Ricotta cheese	1/2 cup	6	Ginger Root	1 Tbsp. Raw	1
Swiss cheese	1 oz	1	Green Bell Peppers	1/2 cup raw	3
Yogurt, low-fat	1 cup	17	Iceberg Lettuce	1-1/2 cups raw	3
Yogurt, fat-free	1 cup	18	Mushrooms	1/2 cup cooked	4
			Okra	1/2 cup cooked	6

*Note : All Carbs are in Grams.

______________________By_Mr._Hitesh_Andel______________________

Chapter 4: Fat

Meaning

Our body needs us to consume fat in order to work properly. Fat comes from a variety of food groups, particularly the milk, meat, and oils food groups. It can also be found in many fried foods, baked goods, and pre-packaged foods.

Fat helps the body absorb vitamin A, vitamin D and vitamin E. These vitamins are fat-soluble, which means they can only be absorbed with the help of fats. It is also important for proper growth, and for keeping you healthy.

A completely fat-free diet would not be healthy, yet it is important that fat be consumed in moderation. A small amount of fat is an essential part of a healthy, balanced diet. Fat is a source of essential fatty acids, which the body cannot make itself.

It is important to keep in mind that fat has the most calories compared to any other nutrient. Controlling fat intake is one of the most important steps in losing or maintaining weight and preventing or delaying type 2 diabetes.

Fat and oil are high in calories. When eating the same amount of fat and carbohydrate or protein, the fat we eat gives us double the amount of calories (9kcal per gram) compared to that of carbohydrate or protein (4kcal per gram).

The body uses fat as a fuel source, and fat is the major storage form of energy in the body. Fat also has many other important functions in the body, and a moderate amount is needed in the diet for good health.

Fats in food come in several forms, including saturated, monounsaturated, and polyunsaturated. Too much fat or too much of the wrong type of fat can be unhealthy.

Fat is often added during cooking or in the preparation of food products. It is one of the main parts of a complete diet and provides energy to the body.

Some examples of foods that contain fats are butter, oil, nuts, meat, fish, and some dairy products.

Types

Fats are nutrients that give you energy. Fats have 9 calories in each gram. Fats help in the absorption of fat-soluble vitamins A, D, E, and K.

Fats are either

- Saturated or
- Unsaturated,

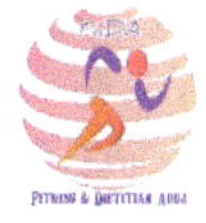

25

☐　Trans

and most foods with fat have both types. But usually there is more of one kind of fat than the other.

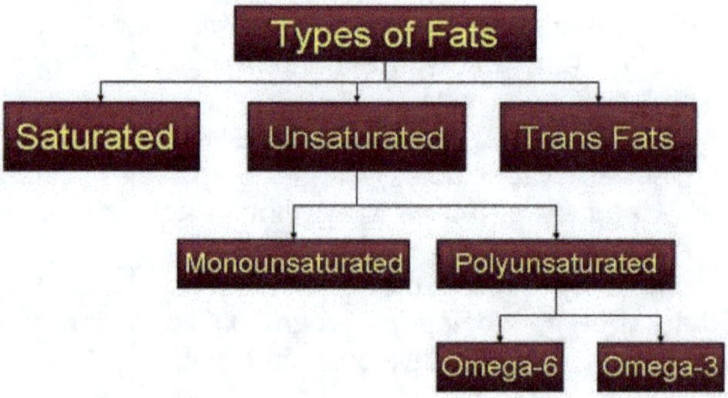

Types of Fats

- Saturated
- Unsaturated
- Trans Fats

Unsaturated → Monounsaturated, Polyunsaturated

Polyunsaturated → Omega-6, Omega-3

Type of Fatty Acid	Found in	Characteristics
Saturated	*Animal fats* (fatty meats, poultry fats and skins) *Dairy products* (butter, cheeses, milk, ice cream)	Tend to remain **solid** at room temperature
Trans	*Fast foods* (deep-fried foods, margarine) *Processed snacks* (packaged cookies, sweets)	
Monounsaturated	*Plant-based foods* (avocado, olives, various nuts) *Oils* (olive oil, canola oil, safflower oils)	Tend to remain **liquid** at room temperature
Polyunsaturated	*Fish* (salmon, tuna, sardines) *Certain vegetables* (dark green, leafy vegetables)	

Saturated fat

Saturated fat is solid at room temperature, which is why it is also known as "solid fat." It is mostly in animal foods, such as milk, cheese, and meat. Poultry and fish have less saturated fat than red meat. Saturated fat is also in tropical oils, such as coconut oil, palm oil, and cocoa butter. You'll find tropical oils in many snacks and in non-dairy foods, such as coffee creamers and whipped toppings. Foods made

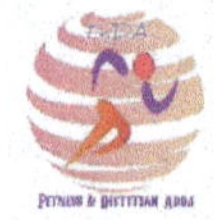

26

with butter, margarine, or shortening (cakes, cookies, and other desserts) have a lot of saturated fat. Saturated fat can raise your cholesterol.

Trans fat

This is a fat that has been changed by a process called hydrogenation. This process increases the shelf life of fat and makes the fat harder at room temperature. Some animal-based foods have small amounts of naturally occurring trans fats. Most trans fat comes from partially hydrogenated oils (PHOs). PHOs cannot be used in food sold in Canada. *Trans fat can raise your cholesterol, so eat as little trans fat as possible.*

Unsaturated fat

Unsaturated fat is liquid at room temperature. It is mostly in oils from plants. If you eat unsaturated fat instead of saturated fat, it may help improve your cholesterol levels. Try to eat mostly unsaturated fats. *Monounsaturated fat and polyunsaturated fat* are types of unsaturated fat.

- **Monounsaturated fat:** This fat is in *avocado*, *nuts*, and *vegetable oils*, such as canola, olive, and peanut oils. Eating foods that are high in monounsaturated fats may help lower your "bad" LDL cholesterol. Monounsaturated fats may also keep "good" HDL cholesterol levels high. But eating more unsaturated fat without cutting back on saturated fat may not lower your cholesterol.
- **Polyunsaturated fat:** This type of fat is *mainly in vegetable oils* such as safflower, sunflower, sesame, soybean, and corn oils. Polyunsaturated fat is also the main fat found in seafood. Eating polyunsaturated fat in place of saturated fat may lower LDL cholesterol. The two types of polyunsaturated fats are omega-3 and omega-6 fatty acids.
  - **Omega-3 fatty acids** are found in foods from plants like soybean oil, canola oil, walnuts, and flaxseed. They are also found in fatty fish and shellfish as eicosapentaenoic acid (EPA) and docosahexaenoic acid (DHA). Salmon, anchovies, herring, sardines, Pacific oysters, trout, Atlantic mackerel, and Pacific mackerel are high in EPA and DHA and lower in mercury.
  - **Omega-6 fatty acids** are found mostly in liquid vegetable oils like soybean oil, corn oil, and safflower oil.

Function / Need

Fat is needed to:

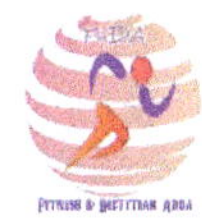

take in and transport fat soluble vitamins A, D, E and K in the body.
- provide essential fatty acids (such as omega 3 and omega 6), which cannot be made by the body.
- protect important organs such as the brain, heart, liver from sudden injury.
- keep the body temperature in the normal range.
- support the different functions of the body.

Tips for Reducing Fat Intake

- Choose low fat dairy products over coconut or full-cream milk.
- Remove any fat that can be seen and skin from poultry. If possible, choose lean meat over fatty meat.
- Replace chicken rice or nasi lemak rice with plain rice.
- Replace roti prata with chapati, dosa or idli.
- Choose steaming, grilling and / or even baking instead of deep-frying when you cook.
- Choose products with a Healthier Choice Symbol - Lower in Saturated Fat.
- Eat All Foods in moderation.
- Taking in more fat than needed will lead to a build-up of additional calories.
- Although monounsaturated and polyunsaturated fats have health advantages, they should be consumed in moderate amounts since all types of fat have the same calorie content.
- A diet high in saturated fat and trans fat tends to raise the level of "bad cholesterol" in the body, which increases the chance of heart disease and stroke.

Fat Deficiency

Reducing your fat intake can be a healthy choice, especially if you currently eat too much fat. However, adopting a **completely fat-free diet is not healthy for most people**. Avoiding fat won't necessarily help you lose weight.

A small amount of fat is an essential part of a healthy, balanced diet. **Fat is a source of essential fatty acids**, which the body cannot make itself. Fat helps the body absorb vitamin A, vitamin D and vitamin E. These vitamins are fat-soluble, which means they can only be absorbed with the help of fats.

If you don't get enough fat in your diet, you may notice symptoms such as dry rashes, hair loss, a weaker immune system, and issues related to vitamin deficiencies. To help maintain good

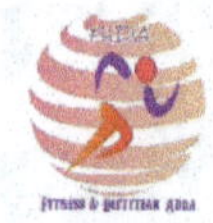

health, most of the fats you eat should be monounsaturated or polyunsaturated fats.

Fat Surplus

Excess consumed energy — usually calories from fats or carbs — is stored in fat cells in the form of triglycerides. This is how your body preserves energy for future needs. Over time, this excess energy results in a fat surplus that can affect your body shape and health.

Surplus dietary fat cannot be converted into other macronutrient forms or excreted, so has to be stored or oxidized. Healthy mammals store excess energy in the form of triacylglycerol (TAG) in lipid droplets within adipocytes rather than oxidizing it, and thus ultimately gain weight.

How does Fat affect us?

Around 25-30% of the total energy you take in should come from fat. For example, for a 2000 kcal diet, the recommended amount of fat you should take in is 55g-65g. Taking in more fat than needed will lead to a build-up of extra calories. If you keep on taking in more calories than you burn through physical activity, you will gain weight and increase your chance of being overweight. The additional fat in your body can increase your risk of getting diabetes, heart disease, high blood pressure and some forms of cancer.

Dietary recommendation

Description	Male	Female
Total Fat	70g	56g
Saturated Fat	Not more than 21g	Not more than 17g
Trans Fat	Not more than 2g*	Not more than 2g*

*This is only a guide and the consumption should be kept to a minimum. A 4g (based on 1,800 - 2,000 kcal diet) increase in trans fat can result in a 23% increase in the risk of heart disease.

Source of Fat

Healthy Fats Source

Omega-3 fatty acids are an especially heart healthy fat and can help with lowering high triglyceride values in your blood.
Omega-3 fats can be found in:

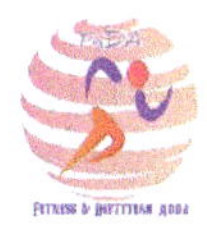

- Fish: salmon, mackerel, herring, sardines, albacore tuna, and rainbow trout
- Tofu and other soybean products
- Walnuts
- Flaxseed and flaxseed oil
- Canola oil

Monounsaturated and polyunsaturated fat are considered "heart healthy" and can help with improving cholesterol when used in place of unhealthy fats.

Some sources of these fats include:

- Avocado
- Nuts and seeds: almonds, cashews, pecans, peanuts, pine nuts, pumpkin, sesame seeds, or sunflower seeds
- Olive oil and olives
- Oils: vegetable oils (such as sunflower, safflower, corn, soybean, and cottonseed)
- Peanut butter

(Source: American Diabetes Association)

Fats to Avoid

Saturated Fats are mainly found in foods that come from animals (such as meat and dairy), but they can also be found in most fried foods and some prepackaged foods.

Saturated fats are unhealthy because they increase LDL ("bad" cholesterol) levels in your body and increase your risk for heart disease. Many saturated fats are "solid" fats that you can see, such as the fat in meat.

Other **sources of saturated fats** include:

- High-fat cheeses
- High-fat cuts of meat
- Whole-fat milk and cream
- Butter
- Ice cream and ice cream products
- Palm and coconut oils

Trans fat is simply liquid oils turned into solid fats during food processing. There is also a small amount of trans fat that occurs naturally in some meat and dairy products, but those found in processed foods tend to be the most harmful to your health. Trans fats serve up a double whammy to your cholesterol, by increasing LDL ("bad" cholesterol) and decreasing HDL ("healthy" cholesterol).

In order to avoid trans fat, look on nutrition labels for ingredients such as "partially hydrogenated" oils or shortening. In

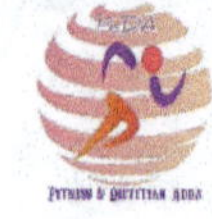

30

addition, look for trans fat in the nutritional information in products, such as commercially baked cookies, crackers, and pies, and fried foods.

Carbs Vs Lipid (Fat)

Carbohydrate (Glycogen)		Lipid (Triglyceride)
Short-term energy storage	**S**torage	Long-term energy storage
More effect on osmotic pressure	**O**smolality	Less effect on osmotic pressure
More readily digested – used for aerobic or anaerobic respiration	**D**igestion	Less easily digested – can only be used for aerobic respiration
Stores half as much ATP per gram (~1760kJ per 100g)	**A**TP Yield	Stores twice as much ATP per gram (~4000kJ per 100g)
Water soluble as monomers / dimers – easier to transport	**S**olubility	Not water soluble (hydrophobic) – more difficult to transport

Here are a few more tips for choosing the best types of fat :-

- Choose leaner cuts of meat that do not have much visible fat.
- Leaner cuts include round cuts and sirloin cuts.
- Trim visible fat off meat before eating.
- Sauté with olive oil or canola oil instead of butter.
- Use olive oil in salad dressings and marinades.
- Use canola oil when baking.
- When reheating soups or stews, skim the solid fats from the top before heating.
- Sprinkle slivered nuts or sunflower seeds on salads instead of bacon bits.
- Snack on a small handful of nuts rather than potato chips or processed crackers.
- Try peanut butter or other nut-butter spreads (which do not contain trans fat) on celery, bananas, or low-fat crackers.
- Add slices of avocado rather than cheese to your sandwich.
- Once or twice a week prepare fish, such as salmon or mackerel, instead of meat.

_______________________By_Mr._Hitesh_Andel_______________________

Chapter 5: Protein

Meaning

Chemically, protein is composed of amino acids, which are organic compounds made of carbon, hydrogen, nitrogen, oxygen or sulfur.

Amino acids are the building blocks of proteins, and proteins are the building blocks of muscle mass, according to *"the National Institutes of Health (NIH)."*

Proteins are large, complex molecules that play many critical roles in the body. They do most of the work in cells and are required for the structure, function, and regulation of the body's tissues and organs.

Your body needs protein to stay healthy and work the way it should. More than 10,000 types are found in everything from your organs to your muscles and tissues to your bones, skin, and hair.

Protein is also a critical part of the processes that fuel your energy and *carry oxygen throughout your body in your blood.*

When we say "protein builds muscle," what we really mean is the body breaks down protein into its amino acids, and those amino acids are synthesized into muscle. Amino acids – the "building blocks of protein" – are compounds that are responsible for a variety of bodily processes, including neurological processes and muscle synthesis. 80% of muscle is made up of amino acids.

When it comes to protein, there are 20 different amino acids that make up each molecule of protein, and these are split into 2 categories:

Non-Essential Amino Acids and **Essential Amino Acids (EAAs)**

- Non-Essential Amino Acids – produced naturally by the body
- Essential Amino Acids – not produced naturally by the body and must be consumed through food or supplementation

Non-essential	Essential	'Conditionally' essential
alanine	valine	cysteine
serine	leucine	tyrosine
asparagine	isoleucine	glutamine
aspartate	methionine	arginine
glutamate	phenylalanine	proline
	threonine	glycine
	lysine	taurine
	histidine	
	tryptophan	

Higher percentages of protein are found in hair, bones, and other organs and tissues with a low water content. Protein molecules are produced in cells by the stepwise alignment of amino acids and are released into the body fluids only after synthesis is complete.

Types of Protein

Two special and common types of proteins are *enzymes and hormones.*

Enzymes, which are produced by living cells, are catalysts in biochemical reactions (like digestion) and are usually complex or conjugated proteins. Each enzyme is specific for the substrate (a reactant that binds to an enzyme) it acts on. The enzyme may help in breakdown, rearrangement, or synthesis reactions.

Enzymes that break down their substrates are called catabolic enzymes, enzymes that build more complex molecules from their substrates are called anabolic enzymes, and enzymes that affect the rate of reaction are called catalytic enzymes.

It should be noted that all enzymes increase the rate of reaction and, therefore, are considered to be organic catalysts. An example of an enzyme is salivary amylase, which hydrolyzes its substrate amylose, a component of starch.

Hormones are chemical-signaling molecules, usually small proteins or steroids, secreted by endocrine cells that act to control or regulate specific physiological processes, including growth, development, metabolism, and reproduction. For example, insulin is a protein hormone that helps to regulate the blood glucose level.

Type	Examples	Functions
Digestive Enzymes	Amylase, lipase, pepsin, trypsin	Help in digestion of food by catabolizing nutrients into monomeric units
Transport	Hemoglobin, albumin	Carry substances in the blood or lymph throughout the body
Structural	Actin, tubulin, keratin	Construct different structures, like the cytoskeleton
Hormones	Insulin, thyroxine	Coordinate the activity of different body systems
Defense	Immunoglobulins	Protect the body from foreign pathogens
Contractile	Actin, myosin	Effect muscle contraction
Storage	Legume storage proteins, egg white (albumin)	Provide nourishment in early development of the embryo and the seedling

33

Categories of Protein

There are two main categories (or sources) of proteins – animal and plant based.

Animal proteins include:

- Whey (dairy)
- Casein (dairy)
- Egg
- Beef
- Chicken etc

Plant Based proteins include:

- Soy
- Pea
- Brown Rice
- Chickpea etc.

The main difference between animal and plant proteins is their amino acid profile. Most animal proteins are complete proteins, meaning they contain all 9 of the essential amino acids (EAAs). Most plant proteins are considered incomplete proteins, meaning they are missing at least one essential amino acid. However, eating multiple plant proteins together can create the effect of complete proteins.

Animal proteins, such as whey protein, have been studied extensively clinically to determine their effect on skeletal muscle and tissue repair so are recommended for athletes and people who need to increase muscle health and mass, like the elderly or post-surgical patients.

There are two main reasons for this. First, whey is a complete protein, meaning that it contains all of the essential amino acids. Secondly, whey proteins are abundant in Branched Chain Amino Acids (BCAAs) which are a subset of EAAs that support muscle growth.

Function of Protein

1. Reduces Appetite and Hunger Levels :

The three macronutrients — fats, carbs, and protein — affect your body in different ways. Studies show that protein is by far the most filling. It helps you feel more full — with less food.

2. Increases Muscle Mass and Strength :

Protein is the building block of your muscles. Therefore, eating adequate amounts of protein helps you maintain your muscle mass and promotes muscle growth when you do strength training.

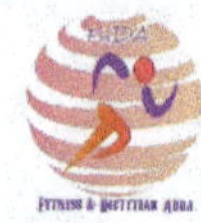

3. Good for Your Bones :

People who eat more protein tend to maintain bone mass better as they age and have a much lower risk of osteoporosis and fractures. This is especially important for women, who are at high risk of osteoporosis after menopause. Eating plenty of protein and staying active is a good way to help prevent that from happening.

4. Reduces Cravings and Desire for Late-Night Snacking :

A food craving is different from normal hunger. It is not just about your body needing energy or nutrients but your brain needing a reward. Yet, cravings can be incredibly hard to control. The best way to overcome them may be to prevent them from occurring in the first place.

One of the best prevention methods is to increase your protein intake. One study in overweight men showed that increasing protein to 25% of calories reduced cravings by 60% and the desire to snack at night by half.

5. Boosts Metabolism and Increases Fat Burning :

Eating can boost your metabolism for a short while. That's because your body uses calories to digest and make use of the nutrients in foods. This is referred to as the thermic effect of food (TEF).

However, not all foods are the same in this regard. In fact, protein has a much higher thermic effect than fat or carbs — 20–35% compared to 5–15%.

High protein intake has been shown to significantly boost metabolism and increase the number of calories you burn. This can amount to 80–100 more calories burned each day.

6. Lowers Your Blood Pressure :

High blood pressure is a major cause of heart attacks, strokes, and chronic kidney disease.

Interestingly, higher protein intake has been shown to lower blood pressure. One study found that, in addition to lowering blood pressure, a high-protein diet also reduced LDL (bad) cholesterol and triglycerides.

7. Helps Maintain Weight Loss :

Because a high-protein diet boosts metabolism and leads to an automatic reduction in calorie intake and cravings, many people who increase their protein intake tend to lose weight almost instantly

8. Does Not Harm Healthy Kidneys :

Many people wrongly believe that a high protein intake harms your kidneys. However, while high protein intake may harm individuals with kidney problems, it has no relevance to people with healthy

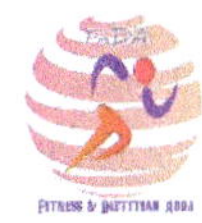

kidneys.It is true that restricting protein intake can benefit people with pre-existing kidney disease. This should not be taken lightly, as kidney problems can be very serious

9. Helps Your Body Repair Itself After Injury :

Protein can help your body repair after it has been injured. This makes perfect sense, as it forms the main building blocks of your tissues and organs.

10. Helps You Stay Fit as You Age :

Eating more protein is one of the best ways to reduce age-related muscle deterioration and prevent sarcopenia.

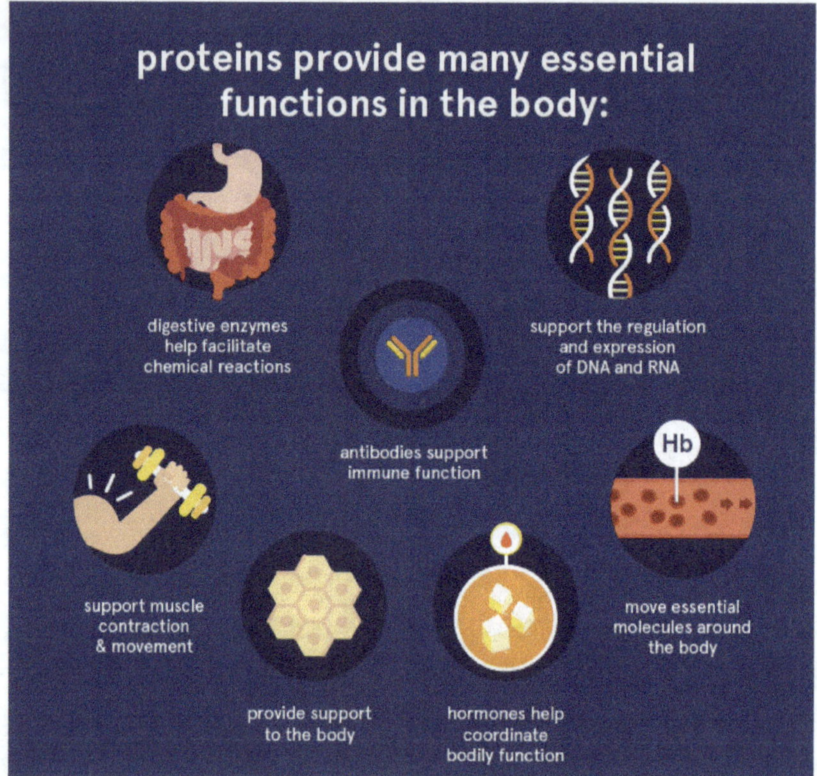

So what if I am vegan or lactose intolerant?

By supplementing your plant protein intake with additional amino acids (e.g. BCAAs) either through other plant protein sources or nutritional supplements, you can get the amino acid levels your body needs for optimal muscle protein synthesis.

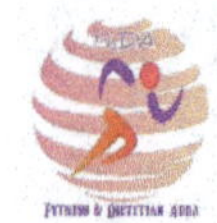

36

For example, lysine, methionine and tryptophan (essential amino acids) are in very low quantities in plant based proteins and therefore you need to supplement to get them into your body to stimulate muscle protein synthesis.

How much protein do I need?

The prevailing research says that you should strive to consume 1 gram per kilogram (1kg = 2.2 lbs for Americans) of bodyweight per day.

This guideline will vary based on your goals. For example, if you are looking to put on muscle, you should increase your protein intake to 2-3 grams per kilogram.

However, protein is not only important for bodybuilders. If you are recovering from an injury or surgery, your body will be in a higher metabolic state and require more energy and tissue building nutrients, so you will want to increase your protein consumption to support the healing process.

Protein is also very important as we age. Beginning around the age of 40, you begin to lose up to 3-5% of your muscle mass per decade, a condition known as *sarcopenia*. Sarcopenia is the reason why falls and fractures are so common among the elderly. Increasing your protein intake, as well as continuing to exercise, can help preserve muscle and fight off sarcopenia.

Age	Protein RDA
child aged 1–3	13 g
child aged 4–8	19 g
child aged 9–13	34 g
female teen aged 14–18	46 g
male teen aged 14–18	52 g
female adult aged 19+	46 g
male adult aged 19+	56 g

Who needs the most protein?

Athletes with high training volumes: Highly active people, those training more than 3 times per week, CrossFitters, competitive athletes, bodybuilders, anyone who's doing a lot of glycolytic activity will perform, recover and feel better on a high protein diet.

Where Does All This Protein Go?

While consuming sufficient protein is important, the truly important metric is not how much we consume, but how much of the

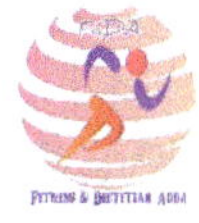

37

protein our muscles actually absorb. Research shows that the average person can *absorb about 10g of protein per hour*, and maxes out at about 30g per meal.

There are certain things we can do to bump up absorption and make sure we get the most out of our protein intake.

1.   Space out Meals:

Intuitively, the first step you can take is to space out your meals and consume appx. 20-30g protein (e.g.100g chicken breast) per meal over multiple meals, instead of eating a few meals of 40-50g protein, since your body will not be able to process that amount of protein at one time.

2.   Try a Protein Complex

A protein complex is a combination of different protein types that have different digestion periods. For example, combining whey (a fast digesting protein) with casein (a slow digesting protein) allows the body to continuously process the protein over a longer period of time than with just whey alone.

3.   Supplement with Digestive Enzymes and HMB

Another option is to increase the absorption rate so that your muscles utilize more of the protein you consume.

Research shows that digestive enzymes like *protease* and *papain* help your body break down protein more efficiently to allow for easier absorption.

Another nutrient that has been shown to increase protein synthesis is HMB (β-Hydroxy β-methylbutyric acid), which is a natural substance used by people ranging from elite athletes looking to put on muscle, to cancer patients suffering from muscle wasting that are hoping to preserve muscle. HMB also has shown to reduce muscle catabolism, meaning you lose less and hold onto more muscle.

High-protein foods

Some high-protein **meats** include:

- Top or bottom round steak (23 grams of protein per 3-ounce serving)
- Lean ground beef (18 grams per 3-ounce serving)
- Pork chops (26 grams per 3-ounce serving)
- Skinless chicken breast (24 grams per 3-ounce serving)
- Turkey breast (24 grams per 3-ounce serving)
- Sockeye salmon (23 grams per 3-ounce serving)
- Yellowfin tuna (25 grams per 3-ounce serving)

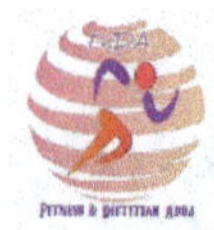

High-protein **dairy foods** include:

- Greek yogurt (23 grams per 8-ounce serving)
- Cottage cheese (14 grams per half-cup serving)
- Eggs (6 grams per large egg)
- 2 percent milk (8 grams per cup)

Some other **high-protein foods** are:

- Some canned foods, like sardines, anchovies and tuna average around 22 grams of protein per serving
- Lentils (13 grams per quarter-cup)
- Peanut butter (8 grams per 2 tablespoons)
- Mixed nuts (6 grams per 2-ounce serving)
- Quinoa (8 grams per 1-cup serving)
- Edamame (8 grams per half-cup serving)
- Soba noodles -Japanese (12 grams per 3-ounce serving)

Complete or ideal proteins

People can produce some amino acids, but must get others from food. The nine amino acids that humans cannot produce on our own are called essential amino acids, according to the NIH. Essential amino acids are: *histidine, isoleucine, leucine, lysine, methionine, phenylalanine, threonine, tryptophan and valine*.

Protein foods that contain all essential amino acids are called complete proteins, according to Crandall. They are also sometimes called ideal proteins or high-quality proteins. Complete proteins include *meat and dairy products, quinoa, hemp seeds, chia seeds and soy*.

Many plant-based proteins are not complete proteins. These include beans, grains and legumes as well as vegetables, which contain small amounts of protein.

Why do we need protein after a workout?

When working out, you put your muscles through a lot. The more strenuous the exercise, the more your muscles will likely need to recover over time. While rest and consistency in workouts are a great way to build upon your progress and make your body stronger, you can help things along with a certain diet. Specifically, protein after a workout is a great way to strengthen your body and your muscles. No matter the type of workout you're doing—something light or something rather active—a meal or snack chocked full or protein is a great choice once you're done.

During your workout, you are actively tearing and breaking apart muscle fibers. This is done to help your muscles grow and get stronger, but it can take a serious toll on the body over time.

Exercise supports muscle growth, but the body can only build upon existing muscles if they recover after each workout. Consuming protein after exercise **helps the muscles to heal and prevents the loss of lean mass**. Lean mass contributes to a muscular and toned appearance.

As discussed, protein is good for building up tissues and fibers, making them stronger and increasing elasticity over time. Due to this, eating protein after a workout actually increases the impact of exercise while also helping to repair muscles, maintain them, and push them to grow.

Those who are exercising regularly but find they aren't building any muscle can chalk this up to a low-protein diet.

The body is also continually breaking down proteins just as part of everyday bodily functions. With this in mind, including a good amount of protein in your diet should always be a necessity.

How to get more protein in your diet ?

The type of protein you eat after a workout isn't as important as providing your body with protein. This means that whether you're eating a hard-boiled egg or drinking a glass of chocolate milk, it doesn't really matter to your muscles. Whatever foods you choose, a good rule of thumb is to provide *only 10-20 grams of protein for your muscles.* Too much protein can become a problem, so be careful.

Of course, the type of protein you consume does matter to the rest of your diet, especially if you're trying to lose fat while you build muscle.

A great protein-packed diet that won't disrupt your progress could consist of the following post-workout snacks:

- **Whey Protein:** Whey protein is a popular option because it digests quickly, provides a good amount of amino acids, and is the recommended 20 grams of protein. Add whey protein to a shake with other ingredients such as peanut butter and bananas for a refreshing on the go protein-recharge.

- **Nutrition Bars:** Nutrition bars are another great option because they come with carbs, sugars, and healthy fats to help your body recharge. Depending upon the vigor of your workout, simple protein is not enough. Carbohydrates, sodium, sugar, and more are needed to give your body much of what it has lost during the workout. Nutrition bars with cocoa, berries, oats, and nuts are all great choices.

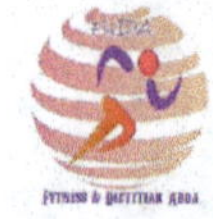

- **Meat, Cheese, and Fruit:** Lean meats and cheeses are a great way to add protein to your body after a workout. There are actually convenient protein packs that come with lean meats like chicken, turkey, or bacon bits, cheese, and fruit or nuts to provide a quick burst of energy when you need it.
- **Rice Cakes:** Rice cakes are a versatile snack that can add some protein to your diet easily and efficiently. Add peanut butter, bananas, berries, or even yogurt on top to make a tasty treat that's also healthy and lean.

What If you take Surplus Protein

Excess protein consumed is usually stored as fat, while the surplus of amino acids is excreted. This can lead to weight gain over time, especially if you consume too many calories while trying to increase your protein intake.

Protein Deficiency

A lack of protein can make you lose muscle mass, which in turn cuts your strength, makes it harder to keep your balance, and slows your metabolism. It can also lead to anemia, when your cells don't get enough oxygen, which makes you tired.

Protein deficiency can arise if a person has a health condition, including:

- an eating disorder, such as anorexia nervosa
- certain genetic conditions
- advanced stages of cancer
- difficulty absorbing nutrients due to a health issue such as irritable bowel syndrome (IBS) or gastric bypass surgery
- Trusted Source

Very low protein intake can lead to:

- weak muscle tone
- edema or swelling due to fluid retention
- thin, brittle hair
- skin lesions
- in adults, a loss of muscle mass
- in children, growth deficits
- hormone imbalances

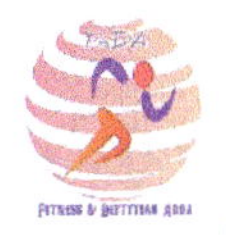

Protein energy Malnutrition Delay in wound healing. Still Birth, Premature Baby. Increased susceptibility to infection. Anemia. Mental retardation. Functions: Helps to build new cells, maintaining or repairing the injured one. Helps to synthesize antibodies, Enzymes & coenzymes hormones etc. Produce Energy.

________________By_Mr._Hitesh_Andel________________

Chapter 6: Vitamins and Minerals

Meaning of Vitamin

Vitamins are substances that our bodies need to develop and function normally. They include vitamins A, C, D, E, and K, choline, and the B vitamins (thiamin, riboflavin, niacin, pantothenic acid, biotin, vitamin B6, vitamin B12, and folate/folic acid).

Vitamins and minerals are considered essential nutrients—because acting in concert, they perform hundreds of roles in the body. They **help shore up bones, heal wounds**, and bolster your immune system. They also convert food into energy, and repair cellular damage.

The term vitamin is derived from the word vitamin, which was coined in 1912 by *Polish biochemist Casimir Funk,* who isolated a complex of micronutrients essential to life.

Classification of Vitamins

Vitamins Are two types:

- **Fat soluble** : A, D, E and K Vitamins.
- **Water Soluble**: C (ascorbic acid) B^1 (thiamine), B^2 (riboflavin), B^3 (niacin), B6 (Pyridoxine) : B12 (Cobalamin), Pantothenic acid, and folic acid.

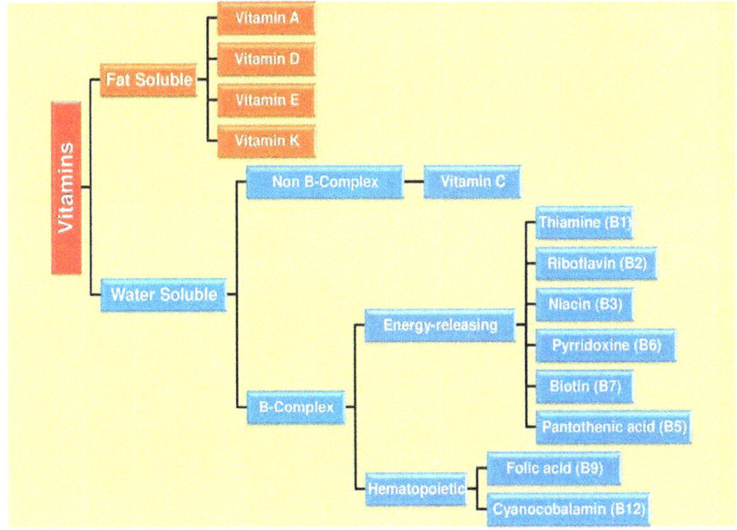

Source of Vitamins
Grains

Whole-grain foods are low in fat. They're also high in fiber and complex carbohydrates. This helps you feel full longer and prevents overeating.

For example, "whole wheat flour" or "whole oat flour." Look for products that have at least 3 grams of fiber per serving. Some enriched flours have fiber, but are not nutrient-rich.

Choose these foods:

- Rolled or steel cut oats.
- Whole-wheat pasta.
- Whole-wheat tortillas.
- Whole-grain (wheat or rye) crackers, breads, and rolls.
- Brown or wild rice.
- Barley, quinoa, buckwheat, whole corn, and cracked wheat.

Fruits and vegetables

Fruits and vegetables naturally are low in fat. They add nutrients, flavor, and variety to your diet. Look for colorful fruits and vegetables, especially orange and dark green.

Choose these foods:

- Broccoli, cauliflower, and Brussels sprouts.
- Leafy greens, such as chard, cabbage, romaine, and bok choy.
- Dark, leafy greens, such as spinach and kale.
- Squash, carrots, sweet potatoes and pumpkin.
- Snap peas, green beans, bell peppers, and asparagus.
- Apples, plums, mangos, papaya, pineapple, and bananas.
- Blueberries, strawberries, cherries, pomegranates, and grapes.
- Citrus fruits, such as grapefruits and oranges.
- Peaches, pears, and melons.
- Tomatoes and avocados.

Meat, poultry, fish, and beans

Pork, veal, and lamb

Choose low-fat, lean cuts of meat. Look for the words "round," "loin," or "leg" in their names. Trim outside fat before cooking. Trim any inside, separable fat before eating. Baking, broiling, and roasting are the healthiest ways to prepare these meats. Limit how often you eat

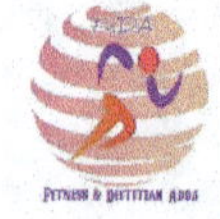

pork, veal, and lamb. Even lean cuts contain more fat and cholesterol compared to other protein sources.

Poultry

Chicken breasts are a good cut of poultry. They are low in fat and high in protein. Remove skin and outside fat before cooking. Baking, broiling, grilling, and roasting are the healthiest ways to prepare poultry.

Fish

Fresh fish and shellfish should be damp and clear in color. They should smell clean and have a firm, springy flesh. If fresh fish isn't available, choose frozen or low-salt canned fish.

Wild-caught oily fish are the best sources of omega-3 fatty acids. This includes salmon, tuna, mackerel, and sardines. Poaching, steaming, baking, and broiling are the healthiest ways to prepare fish.

Choose these foods:
- Wild-caught salmon and other oily fish.
- Haddock and other white fish.
- Wild-caught tuna (canned or fresh).
- Shrimp, mussels, scallops, and lobster (without added fat).

Beans and other non-meat sources

Non-meat sources of protein also can be nutrient-rich. Try a serving of beans, peanut butter, other nuts, or seeds.

Choose these foods:
- Legumes, such as beans, lentils, and chickpeas.
- Seeds and nuts, including nut butters.

Dairy and dairy substitutes

Choose skim milk, low-fat milk, or enriched milk substitutes. Try replacing cream with evaporated skim milk in recipes and coffee. Choose low-fat or fat-free cheeses.

Choose these foods:
- Low-fat, skim, nut, or enriched milk, like soy or rice.
- Skim ricotta cheese in place of cream cheese.
- Low-fat cottage cheese.
- String cheese.
- Plain nonfat yogurt in place of sour cream.

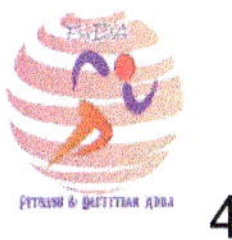

What happens if we take Surplus Vitamins?

Hypervitaminosis is a condition of abnormally high storage levels of vitamins, which can lead to various symptoms such as over excitement, irritability, or even toxicity.

Generally, toxic levels of vitamins stem from high supplement intake and not always from natural sources but rather the mix of natural, derived vitamins and enhancers (vitamin boosters).

Function of Vitamins

Type of Vitamin	Function	Examples of Ingrendients
Vitamin A	Vision and cell development in the body	Sweet potato, mangoes, eggs
Vitamin B1	Energy metabolism and nervous system function	Tuna, whole grains, pork
Vitamin B2	Energy metabolism and normal vision	Mushrooms, whole grains, milk
Vitamin B3	Energy metabolism	Whole grains, milk, eggs, meat
Vitamin B5	Energy metabolism	Mushrooms, avocado, beef, poultry
Vitamin B6	Synthesis in new cells	Green leafy vegetables, fruits, fish
Vitamin B7	Energy metabolism	Nuts, egg yolk, liver, fish
Vitamin B9	Synthesis in new cells	Green leafy vegetables, legumes, liver
Vitamin B12	Synthesis in new cells	Lamb, oysters, sardines
Vitamin C	Immunity and formation of collagen in skin	Citrus fruits, strawberries, tomatoes, potatoes
Vitamin D	Maintains calcium and phosphorus in blood	Fatty fish, fish liver oils, eggs
Vitamin E	Antioxidant	Nuts, green leafy vegetables, fish
Vitamin K	Blood clotting	Spinach, green leafy vegetables

46

Deficiency of Vitamins

Vitamin Deficiency Symptoms Chart		
Vitamin	**Deficiency Symptoms**	**Where to Find It**
A	Dry eyes & skin; Increased infections; Issues with sight, Dry hair, Broken fingernails, Pruritus	Liver and other organ meats; salmon; green, leafy vegetables; orange and yellow vegetables; fruits, including apricots, and mangos; dairy products
B1 (thiamine)	Fatigue; Irritability; Beriberi	Whole grains; meat (especially pork); fish; legumes; seeds; nuts
B2 (riboflavin)	Cracks in corners of the mouth; Dry patches on the head	Cheese; almonds; lamb; mackerel; eggs; pork; mushrooms; sesame seeds; spinach
B3 (niacin)	Mental confusion and dementia; Scaly skin; Muscle weakness; Diarrhea; Memory impairment; Disorientation; Depression; Delirium, mania, or paranoia	Dairy; eggs; enriched bread and cereal; fish; lean meat; legumes; nuts
B5 (Pantothenic acid)	Seizures; Scaly rash; Red tongue; Cracks in corner of mouth; Pins-and-needles sensation in hands and feet	Avocado; broccoli; kale; cabbage; eggs, legumes; milk; mushrooms; organ meat; poultry; potatoes; yeast
B12 (cobala min)	Fatigue; Anemia; Paleness; Weakness; Shortness of breath; Dizziness; Tingling or loss of sensation in hands and feet; Confusion and dementia	Clams; liver; fortified breakfast cereal; trout; salmon; tuna; haddock; milk
Folate	Fatigue; Anemia; Paleness; Shortness of breath and dizziness; Red and sore tongue; Reduced sense of taste; Weight loss; Depression	Beans; lentils; spinach; asparagus; lettuce; avocado; broccoli; mango; oranges

C	Bleeding gums; Infection; Dry hair and skin; Gingivitis; Nosebleeds; Weight gain, Painful joints; Weakened tooth enamel	Citrus fruits; peppers; guava; kale; broccoli; tomatoes; peas
D	Weak and brittle bones; Bone pain; Muscle weakness	Cod liver oil; swordfish; salmon; tuna; orange juice; milk; yogurt; sardines; liver; eggs

Minerals

A mineral is a naturally occurring inorganic solid, with a definite chemical composition, and an ordered atomic arrangement. This may seem a bit of a mouthful, but if you break it down it becomes simpler. Minerals are naturally occurring.

Minerals are those elements on the earth and in foods that our bodies need to develop and function normally. Those essential for health include *calcium, phosphorus, potassium, sodium, chloride, magnesium, iron, zinc, iodine, chromium, copper, fluoride, molybdenum, manganese, and selenium.*

Minerals; we need in daily life

Macro minerals (> 100 mg/day)*	Micro minerals (<100 mg/day)*
Calcium	Iron
Phosphorus	Zinc
Magnesium	Copper
Sulfur	Iodine
Sodium*	Fluoride
Potassium*	Manganese
Chloride*	Selenium
	Chromium
	Molybdenum

Classification of Minerals

Classification of Minerals

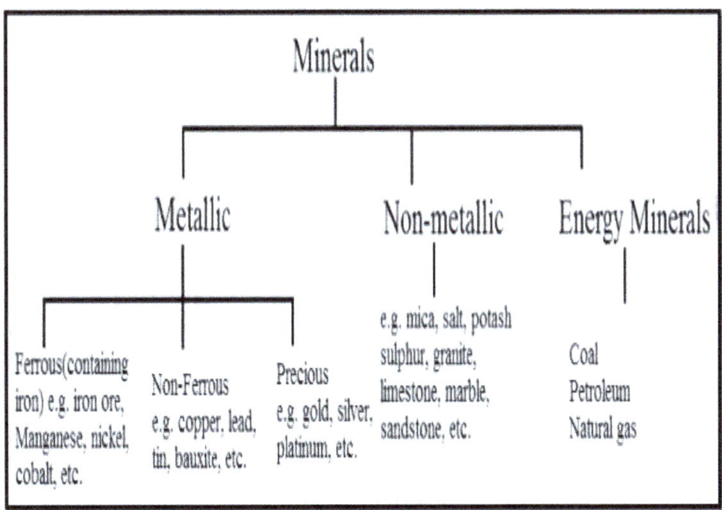

Source and Function of Minerals

Macro minerals

Mineral	Function	Sources
Sodium	Needed for proper fluid balance, nerve transmission, and muscle contraction	Table salt, soy sauce; large amounts in processed foods; small amounts in milk, breads, vegetables, and unprocessed meats
Chloride	Needed for proper fluid balance, stomach acid	Table salt, soy sauce; large amounts in processed foods; small amounts in milk, meats, breads, and vegetables

49

Potassium	Needed for proper fluid balance, nerve transmission, and muscle contraction	Meats, milk, fresh fruits and vegetables, whole grains, legumes
Calcium	Important for healthy bones and teeth; helps muscles relax and contract; important in nerve functioning, blood clotting, blood pressure regulation, immune system health	Milk and milk products; canned fish with bones (salmon, sardines); fortified tofu and fortified soy milk; greens (broccoli, mustard greens); legumes
Phosphorus	Important for healthy bones and teeth; found in every cell; part of the system that maintains acid-base balance	Meat, fish, poultry, eggs, milk, processed foods (including soda pop)
Magnesium	Found in bones; needed for making protein, muscle contraction, nerve transmission, immune system health	Nuts and seeds; legumes; leafy, green vegetables; seafood; chocolate; artichokes; "hard" drinking water
Sulfur	Found in protein molecules	Occurs in foods as part of protein: meats, poultry, fish, eggs, milk, legumes, nuts

Trace minerals (micro minerals)

The body needs trace minerals in very small amounts. Note that iron is considered to be a trace mineral, although the amount needed is somewhat more than for other micro minerals.

Mineral	Function	Sources
Iron	Part of a molecule (hemoglobin) found in red blood cells that carries oxygen in the body; needed for energy metabolism	Organ meats; red meats; fish; poultry; shellfish (especially clams); egg yolks; legumes; dried fruits; dark, leafy greens; iron-enriched breads and cereals; and fortified cereals
Zinc	Part of many enzymes; needed for making protein and genetic material; has a function in taste perception, wound healing, normal fetal development, production of sperm, normal growth and sexual maturation, immune system health	Meats, fish, poultry, leavened whole grains, vegetables
Iodine	Found in thyroid hormone, which helps regulate growth, development, and metabolism	Seafood, foods grown in iodine-rich soil, iodized salt, bread, dairy products
Selenium	Antioxidant	Meats, seafood, grains
Copper	Part of many enzymes; needed for iron metabolism	Legumes, nuts and seeds, whole grains, organ meats, drinking water
Manganese	Part of many enzymes	Widespread in foods, especially plant foods
Fluoride	Involved in formation of bones and teeth; helps prevent tooth decay	Drinking water (either fluoridated or naturally containing fluoride), fish, and most teas

Chromium	Works closely with insulin to regulate blood sugar (glucose) levels	Unrefined foods, especially liver, brewer's yeast, whole grains, nuts, cheeses
Molybdenum	Part of some enzymes	Legumes; breads and grains; leafy greens; leafy, green vegetables; milk; liver

Other trace nutrients known to be essential in tiny amounts include nickel, silicon, vanadium, and cobalt.

Deficiency of Minerals

There are different types of diets that might result in this deficiency. A poor diet that relies on junk food, or a diet that lacks adequate fruits and vegetables can be possible causes. Alternatively, a very low-calorie diet may produce this deficiency.

This includes people in weight-loss programs or with eating disorders. Older adults with poor appetites may also not get enough calories or nutrients in their diet.

Restricted diets may also cause you to have a mineral deficiency. Vegetarians, vegans, and people with food allergies or lactose intolerance might experience mineral deficiency if they fail to manage their diet effectively.

Difficulty with digestion of food or absorption of nutrients can result in mineral deficiency. Potential causes of these difficulties include:

- diseases of the liver, gallbladder, intestine, pancreas, or kidney
- surgery of the digestive tract
- chronic alcoholism
- medications such as antacids, antibiotics, laxatives, and diuretics

Mineral deficiency can also result from an increased need for certain minerals. Women, for instance, may encounter this need during pregnancy, heavy menstruation, and post menopause.

The symptoms of a mineral deficiency depend upon which nutrient the body lacks. Possible symptoms include:

- constipation, bloating, or abdominal pain
- decreased immune system
- diarrhea
- irregular heart beat
- loss of appetite

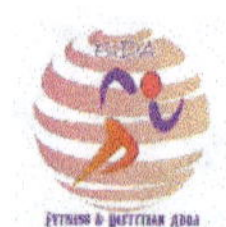

- muscle cramping
- nausea and vomiting
- numbness or tingling in the extremities
- poor concentration
- slow social or mental development in children
- weakness or tiredness

Source of Minerals

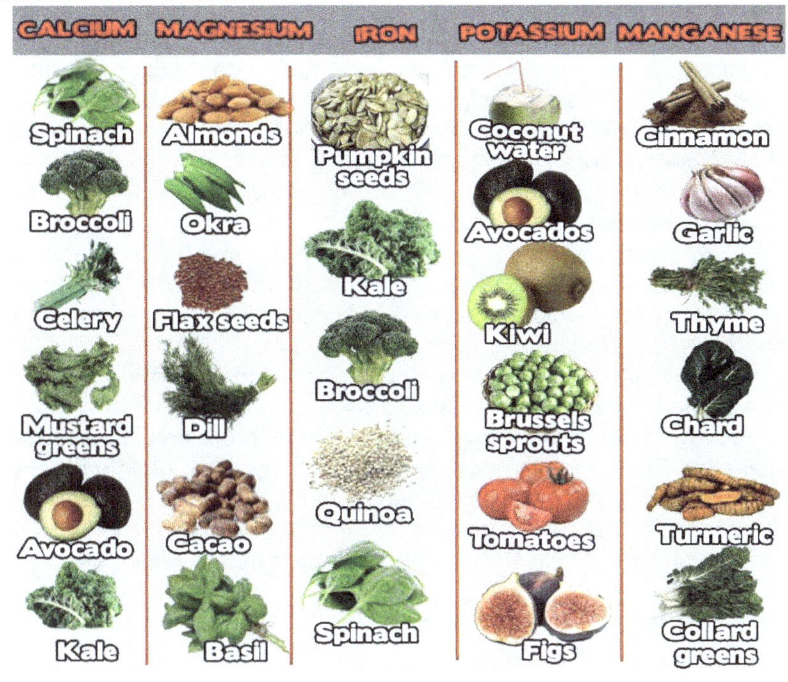

___________________By_Mr._Hitesh_Andel___________________

Chapter 7: Calorie

Meaning of Calorie or Energy

Energy is defined as the capacity to do work. Through the process of digestion, we convert the food we eat to energy. This food energy is calculated as Calories (C) or kilocalories (kcal) or Joules (J).

Food energy is chemical energy that animals (including humans) derive from their food and molecular oxygen through the process of cellular respiration.

The amount of energy in an item of food or drink is measured in calories. Calories in the foods we eat provide energy in the form of heat so that our bodies can function. This means that we need to eat a certain amount of calories just to sustain life. But if we take in too many calories, then we risk gaining weight.

A calorie (Cal, Calorie or kcal) is a unit of measurement — but it doesn't measure weight or length.

A calorie is a unit of measure of energy. When you hear something contains 100 calories, it's a way of describing how much energy your body could get from eating or drinking it. Specifically, it is defined as

"the amount of heat needed to raise the temperature of one gram of water by one degree Celsius."

The amount of energy in an item of food or drink is measured in calories. Energy is provided by the carbohydrate, protein and fat in the food and drinks we consume. It is also provided by alcohol. Different food and drinks provide different amounts of energy. You can find this information on food labels when they are present.

Macronutrient Calories Per Gram

- ☐ **Carbohydrate**: 4 calories per gram
- ☐ **Protein**: 4 calories per gram
- ☐ **Fat**: 9 calories per gram
- ☐ **Alcohol**: 7 calories per gram

Recommended Daily Caloric Intake

The 2020–2025 Dietary Guidelines for Americans indicate that the daily recommended caloric intake for adults can range from 1,600 to 3,200 calories per day. This is a general estimate, as there are many variables to consider when determining an ideal daily caloric intake.

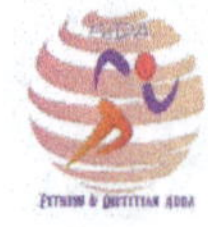

For instance, the calorie needs for males are slightly higher (2,200 to 3,200 calories per day) than the needs for females (1,600 to 2,400 calories daily) according to these guidelines. Your caloric intake also depends on other factors, such as your age, activity level, and metabolism.

The 2020–2025 Dietary Guidelines recommend that your diet be split according to these percentages:

- 10% to 35% protein
- 45% to 65% carbohydrates
- 20% to 35% fat

What are low-calorie and very low-calorie diets?

A low-calorie diet is an eating plan that supplies around 1,200 to 1,500 calories each day while a very low-calorie diet is closer to 800 calories per day. Consuming too few calories can be harmful to your health, so a very low-calorie diet is only recommended when under a doctor's supervision.

A kilocalorie is another word for what's commonly called a calorie, so 1,000 calories will be written as 1,000kcals.

KCAL   VERSUS   CAL

Characteristics	kcal	cal
Size	1	1000
Energy	Amount of energy needed to increase temperature of 1kg of water by 1 °C	Amount of energy needed to increase temperature of 1g of water by 1 °C
Food calorie	Known as the food calorie	Not known as the food calorie
Food labels	Used on food labels, but called a Calorie	Not used on food labels
Metric	kilojoule	joule

Instead, the terms calories — capitalized or not — and kcal are used interchangeably and refer to the same amount of energy in relation to food or energy burned with exercise.

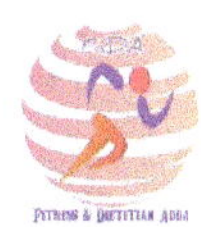

Therefore, you don't need to convert them, as 1 kilocalorie equals 1 calorie in nutrition. Calories may also be expressed as kilojoules (kJ).

Kilojoules are the metric measurement of calories. To find the energy content in kilojoules, multiply the calorie figure by 4.18.

When it comes to nutrition and exercise, kilocalories (kcal) and calories equal the same amount of energy. Calories may also be expressed as kilojoules (kJ), with one calorie or kcal equaling 4.18 kJ.

Below is a list of countries and which label they use for energy :

- <u>India</u> : Kcal and calories both
- United States : calories
- Canada : calories
- European Union (EU) : kJ and kcal
- Australia and New Zealand : kJ or both kJ and kcal
- China : kJ

Energy Storage Analogy

A calorie is a measure of energy, specifically heat. It's a measurement of an indirect use of your biological fuels. Your body doesn't really convert things to "calories", it converts them to **ATP** which is used as energy.

ATP (Adenosine triphosphate) is the **energy currency** of the cell – in this respect it is same as *cash*

- Cash is earned when you work (*cell respiration*) and can be spent in a number of ways (*metabolism*)
- Storing energy as carbohydrates (i.e. glycogen) is similar to keeping the cash in a *wallet*
- It is easier to carry around (monosaccharides and disaccharides are water soluble)
- It is readily accessible (carbohydrates are easier to digest)
- You cannot carry as much (carbohydrates store less energy per gram)
- Storing energy as lipids (i.e. triglycerides) is similar to keeping the cash in a *safe*
- It is not viable to carry around (triglycerides are insoluble in water)
- It is harder to access (triglycerides cannot be easily digested)
- You can keep more cash in it (triglycerides store more energy per gram)

56

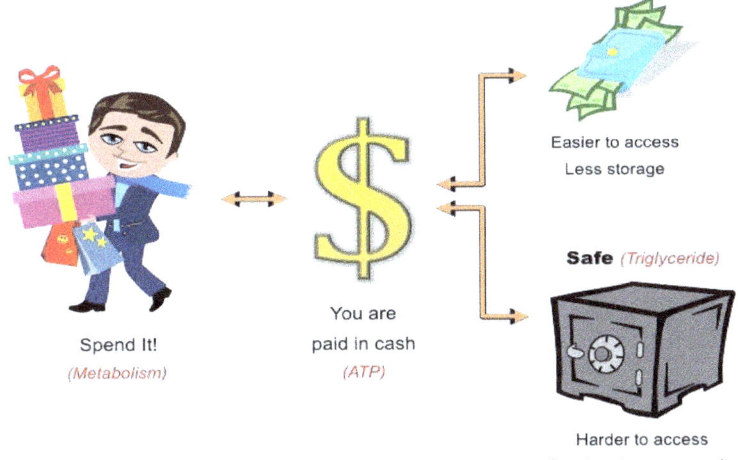

Conversion of Fat into energy

Our bodies use *glucose* all the time because certain tissues, notably the *brain and red blood cells, cannot survive without it*. Blood glucose levels must be maintained all the time, even during starvation. In that case, amino acids from *muscle protein* breakdown serve as a source of carbons for gluconeogenesis, which take place in the *liver*.

"Fat, mobilized from adipose, is the major source of energy."

After a typical mixed meal, carbohydrates are the preferred fuel while *most of the fat is stored in adipose*. Four hours later, fat starts being mobilized from adipose. During the overnight fast, fat is a major source of energy.

If you are maintaining your weight, the amount of carbs and fat you eat are oxidized over a 24 hour cycle.

Scientists have shown that when either lean or obese individuals *exercise after eating a high fat meal, their fats are broken down and oxidized in skeletal muscle, making them healthier*. These results show for the first time how a high fat diet and exercise stimulate the breakdown of fats and may help design ways to reduce excessive fat in the body.

Max Lafontan and colleagues investigated how fat is broken down in both lean and obese subjects who exercised *after either fasting or eating a high-fat diet*. They noticed that after eating a high-fat diet, fats were broken down in both lean and obese individuals. *Under fasting conditions, the breakdown of fats was more pronounced in the lean subjects, but the high fat meal enhanced lipolysis in the obese subjects*

Fat is broken down inside fat cells to generate energy by a process called *lipolysis*. The resulting fatty acids are released into the bloodstream and carried to tissues that require energy. In obese individuals, too much fat accumulates, compromising lipolysis, but the details of how this happens are not well understood. Also, obese individuals can show altered responsiveness to the stress hormones epinephrine and norepinephrine in their subcutaneous fat.

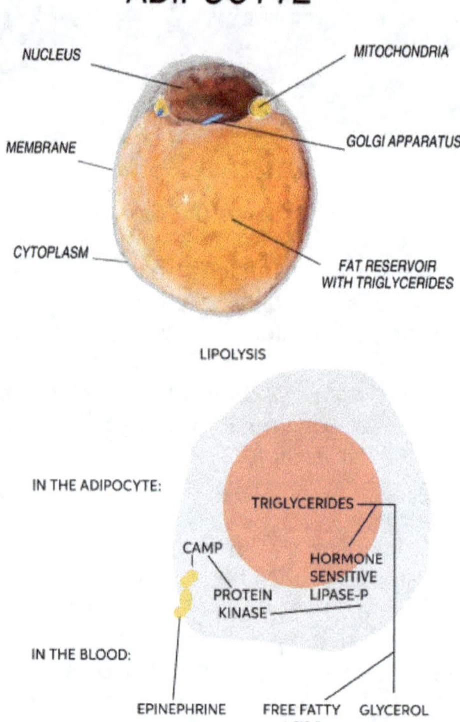

Types of Lipolysis

Lipolysis absorbs or releases fatty acids and glycerol from the cells and helps in maintaining lipid homeostasis and energy.

There are three major functions that occur in vertebrates as part of lipolysis:

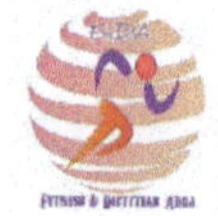

58

- **Gastrointestinal lipolysis** is the one in which breakdown and absorption of dietary triglycerides (also known as triacylglycerol) happen. This involves enzymes like lingual, gastric, and pancreatic lipase.
- Vascular lipolysis which is responsible for the hydrolysis of triglycerides that are associated with lipoproteins in the bed of the capillaries. The enzymes that are used for this are lipoprotein lipase and hepatic lipase.

- Intracellular lipolysis helps in the hydrolysis of triglycerides that are stored in the lipid bodies within the cells. This process uses acid and neutral lipases.

Laser Lipolysis

Laser Lipolysis is a kind of cosmetic surgery in which the fats are removed from the body using laser energy. It helps change the shape of the body by targeting fats in the specific parts of the body and removing them.

A person with a lot of fatty tissues in the thighs, abdomen, or hips might choose to get the fats removed from these places after consulting a plastic surgeon. A laser is used to break the fatty cells and reduce its volume. It also helps in tightening the skin by vacuuming out the extra fats in that area. It has a little risk of scarring in the area the laser is used but is safe otherwise.

Though laser lipolysis changes the way the body appears by the removal of fatty tissues, the long-lasting effects of the procedure depend on the diet and exercise. One can gain back the weight in case he/she is not mindful of what he/she eats and the effects of lipolysis can no longer be seen.

Triglycerides

Triacylglycerols (also known as triglycerides) are the molecules that make up animal fats and vegetable oils. They are used as food storage molecules. They are made of four components - a glycerol molecule attached to three fatty acids. This example has palmitic acid, oleic acid, and stearic acid.

_______________________By_Mr._Hitesh_Andel_______________________

Chapter 8: Basics of Diet

Introduction of Diet

The ancient Indians ate a diet of mostly **wheat, barley, legumes, vegetables, fruits** (Indian dates, mangoes, and berries), **meats** (sheep and goats), **dairy products and honey**. Archeologists have found fishing nets and hooks in the ruins of early Indian civilizations, showing that they also liked to catch and eat fish.

Staple foods eaten today include a variety of lentils (dal), whole-wheat flour (aṭṭa), rice, and pearl millet (bājra), which has been cultivated in the Indian subcontinent since 6200 BCE.

Meaning of Diet

The food we normally eat in a day is our diet. For growth and maintenance of good health, our diet should have all the nutrients that our body needs, in the right quantities. Not too much of one and not too little of the other. The diet should also contain a good amount of roughage (fibrous indigestible material) and water. Such a diet is called a balanced diet.

Balanced Diet

A balanced diet is a **diet that contains different kinds of foods in certain quantities and proportions** so that the requirement for calories, proteins, minerals, vitamins and alternative nutrients is adequate and a small provision is reserved for additional nutrients to endure the short length of leanness.

There are seven essential factors for a balanced diet: **carbs, protein, fat, fibre, vitamins, minerals and water**. Fat : 20–35% of total calories, Vitamins & minerals: Trace, Protein: 10–35% of total calories, Carbs: 45–55% of total calories.

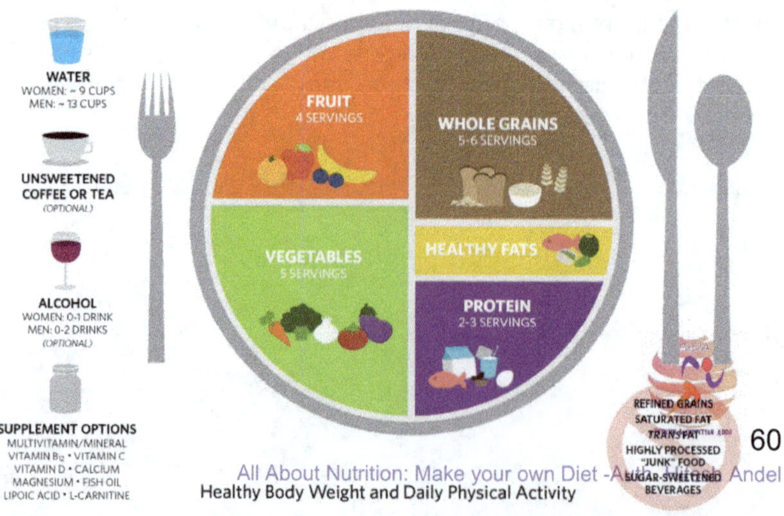

Components of Diet

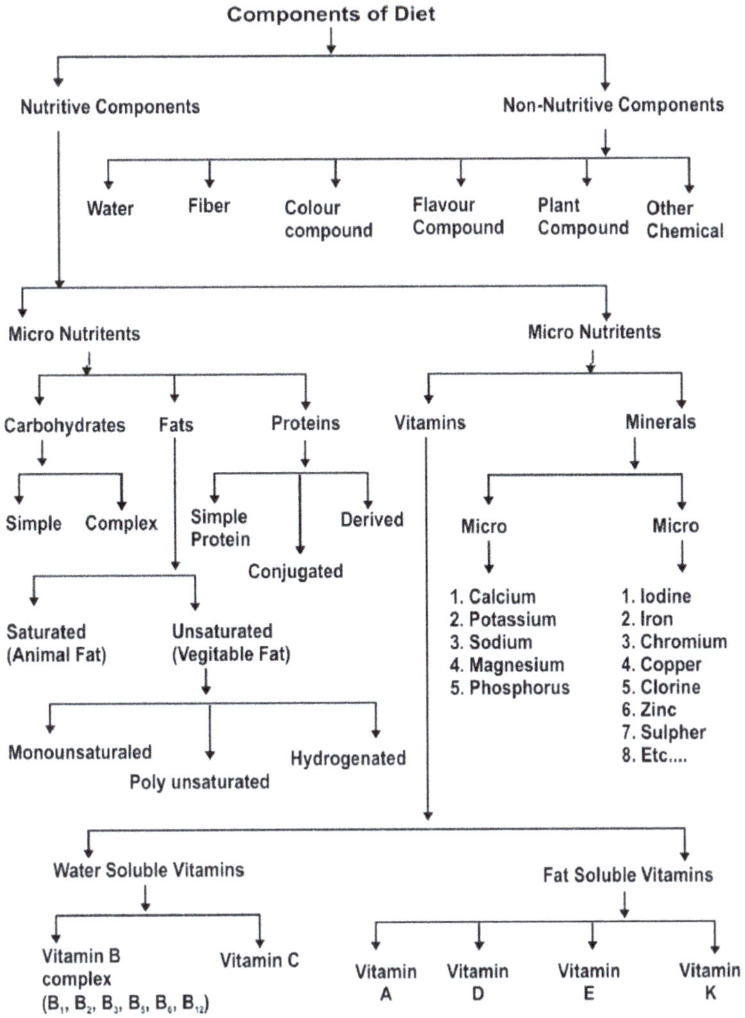

Components of Diet

- **Nutritive Components**
- **Non-Nutritive Components**
  - Water
  - Fiber
  - Colour compound
  - Flavour Compound
  - Plant Compound
  - Other Chemical

Micro Nutritents (under Nutritive Components)

- Carbohydrates
  - Simple
  - Complex
- Fats
  - Simple Protein
  - Conjugated
  - Derived
- Proteins
- Saturated (Animal Fat)
- Unsaturated (Vegitable Fat)
  - Monounsaturaled
  - Poly unsaturated
  - Hydrogenated

Micro Nutritents

- Vitamins
  - Micro
    1. Calcium
    2. Potassium
    3. Sodium
    4. Magnesium
    5. Phosphorus
- Minerals
  - Micro
    1. Iodine
    2. Iron
    3. Chromium
    4. Copper
    5. Clorine
    6. Zinc
    7. Sulpher
    8. Etc....

Water Soluble Vitamins

- Vitamin B complex (B_1, B_2, B_3, B_5, B_6, B_{12})
- Vitamin C

Fat Soluble Vitamins

- Vitamin A
- Vitamin D
- Vitamin E
- Vitamin K

*Already discussed in previous chapters.

Types of Diet

1. The Paleo Diet

The paleo diet claims that you should eat the same foods that your *hunter-gatherer ancestors* ate before agriculture developed.

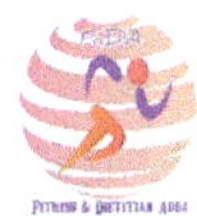

61

The theory is that most modern diseases can be linked to the Western diet and the consumption of grains, dairy, and processed foods.

While it's debatable whether this diet really provides the same foods our ancestors ate, it is linked to several impressive health benefits.

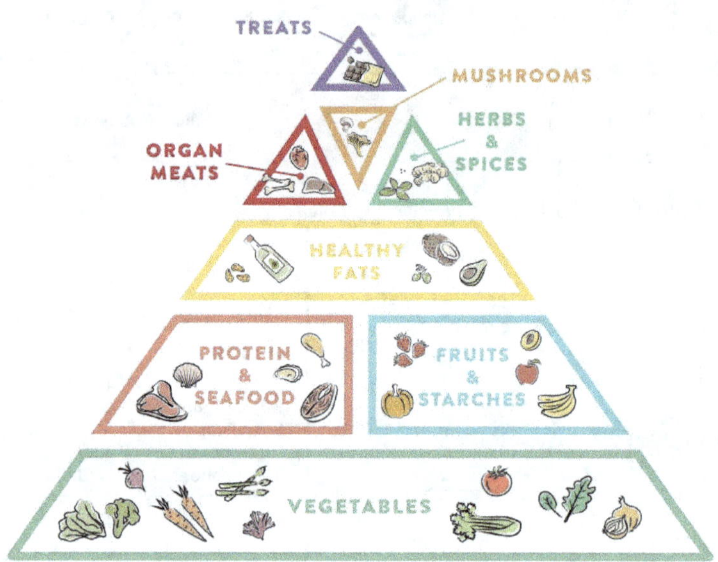

PALEO FOOD PYRAMID

How it works: The paleo diet emphasizes whole foods, lean protein, vegetables, fruits, nuts, and seeds, while discouraging processed foods, sugar, dairy, and grains.

Some more flexible versions of the paleo diet also allow for dairy like cheese and butter, as well as tubers like potatoes and sweet potatoes.

Weight loss: Several studies have shown that the paleo diet can lead to significant weight loss and reduced waist size.

In studies, paleo dieters automatically eat much fewer carbs, more protein, and 300–900 fewer calories per day

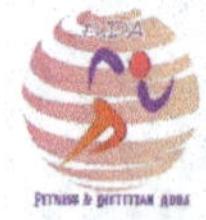

62

Other benefits: The diet seems effective at reducing risk factors for heart disease, such as cholesterol, blood sugar, blood triglycerides, and blood pressure

The drawback: The paleo diet eliminates whole grains, legumes, and dairy, which are healthy and nutritious.

2. The Vegan Diet

The vegan diet _restricts all animal products_ for ethical, environmental, or health reasons.
Veganism is also associated with resistance to animal exploitation and cruelty.

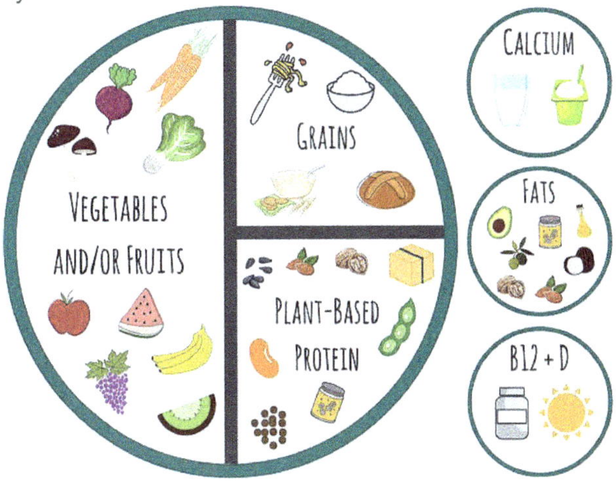

How it works: Veganism is the strictest form of vegetarianism.
 In addition to eliminating meat, it eliminates dairy, eggs, and animal-derived products, such as gelatin, honey, albumin, whey, casein, and some forms of vitamin D3.

Weight loss: A vegan diet seems to be very effective at helping people lose weight — often without counting calories — because its very low fat and high fiber content may make you feel fuller for longer.
 Vegan diets are consistently linked to lower body weight and body mass index (BMI) compared to other diets.
 One 18-week study showed that people on a vegan diet lost 4.2 kg (9.3 pounds) more than those on a control diet. The vegan group was allowed to eat until fullness, but the control group had to restrict calories

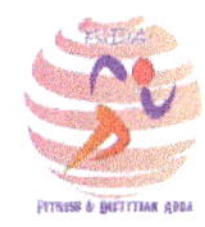

63

Other benefits: Plant-based diets are linked to a reduced risk of heart disease, type 2 diabetes, and premature death.

Limiting processed meat may also reduce your risk of Alzheimer's disease and dying from heart disease or cancer.

The drawback: Because vegan diets eliminate animal foods completely, they may be low in several nutrients, including vitamin B12, vitamin D, iodine, iron, calcium, zinc, and omega-3 fatty acids.

3. Low-Carb Diet

Low-carb diets have been popular for decades — especially for weight loss. There are several types of low-carb diets, but all involve *limiting carb intake* to 20–150 grams per day.

The primary aim of the diet is to force your body to use more fats for fuel instead of using carbs as a main source of energy.

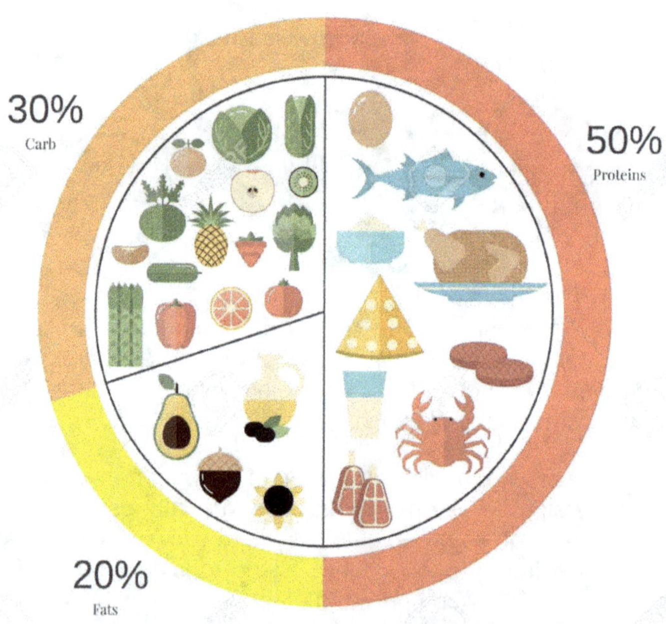

How it works: Low-carb diets emphasize unlimited amounts of protein and fat while severely limiting your carb intake.

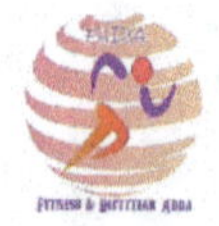

64

When carb intake is very low, fatty acids are moved into your blood and transported to your liver, where some of them are turned into *ketones*.

Your body can then use fatty acids and ketones in the absence of carbs as its primary energy source.

Weight loss: Numerous studies indicate that low-carb diets are extremely helpful for weight loss, especially in overweight and obese individuals.

They seem to be very effective at reducing dangerous belly fat, which can become lodged around your organs.

People on very low-carb diets commonly reach a state called ketosis. Many studies note that ketogenic diets lead to more than twice the weight loss than a low-fat, calorie-restricted diet.

Other benefits: Low-carb diets tend to reduce your appetite and make you feel less hungry, leading to an automatic reduction in calorie intake.

Furthermore, low-carb diets may benefit many major disease risk factors, such as blood triglycerides, cholesterol levels, blood sugar levels, insulin levels, and blood pressure.

The drawback: Low-carb diets do not suit everyone. Some feel great about them while others feel miserable. Some people may experience an increase in "bad" LDL cholesterol. In extremely rare cases, very low-carb diets can cause a serious condition called nondiabetic ketoacidosis. This condition seems to be more common in lactating women and can be fatal if left untreated.

However, low-carb diets are safe for the majority of people.

4. The Ultra-Low-Fat Diet

An ultra-low-fat diet restricts your _consumption of fat to under 10% of daily calories_. Generally, a low-fat diet provides around 30% of its calories as fat. Studies reveal that this diet is ineffective for weight loss in the long term.

Proponents of the ultra-low-fat diet claim that traditional low-fat diets are not low enough in fat and that fat intake needs to stay under 10% of total calories to produce health benefits and weight loss.

How it works: An ultra-low-fat diet contains 10% or fewer calories from fat. The diet is mostly plant-based and has a limited intake of

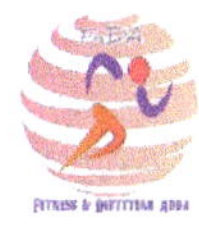

65

animal products. Therefore, it's generally very high in carbs — around 80% of calories — and low in protein — at 10% of calories.

Weight loss: This diet has proven very successful for weight loss among obese individuals. In one study, obese individuals lost an average of 140 pounds (63 kg) on an ultra-low-fat diet.

Another 8-week study with a diet containing 7–14% fat showed an average weight loss of 14.8 pounds (6.7 kg).

Other benefits: Studies suggest that ultra-low-fat diets can improve several risk factors for heart disease, including high blood pressure, high cholesterol, and markers of inflammation. Surprisingly, this high-carb, low-fat diet can also lead to significant improvements in type 2 diabetes.

Furthermore, it may slow the progression of multiple sclerosis — an autoimmune disease that affects your brain, spinal cord, and optic nerves in the eyes.

The drawback: The fat restriction may cause long-term problems, as fat plays many important roles in your body. These include helping build cell membranes and hormones, as well as helping your body absorb fat-soluble vitamins.

Moreover, an ultra-low-fat diet limits intake of many healthy foods, lacks variety, and is extremely hard to stick to.

5. The Atkins Diet

The Atkins diet is the most well-known *low-carb weight loss diet*. Its proponents insist that you can lose weight by eating as much protein and fat as you like, as long as you avoid carbs.

The main reason why low-carb diets are so effective for weight loss is that they reduce your appetite.This causes you to eat fewer calories without having to think about it.

How it works: The Atkins diet is split into four phases. It starts with an induction phase, during which you *eat under 20 grams of carbs per day for two weeks.*

The other phases involve slowly reintroducing healthy carbs back into your diet as you approach your goal weight.

Weight loss: The Atkins diet has been studied extensively and found to lead to faster weight loss than low-fat diets.

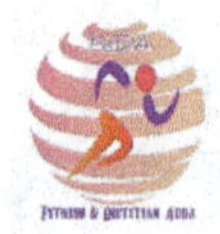

Other studies note that low-carb diets are very helpful for weight loss. They are especially successful in reducing belly fat, the most dangerous fat that lodges itself in your abdominal cavity.

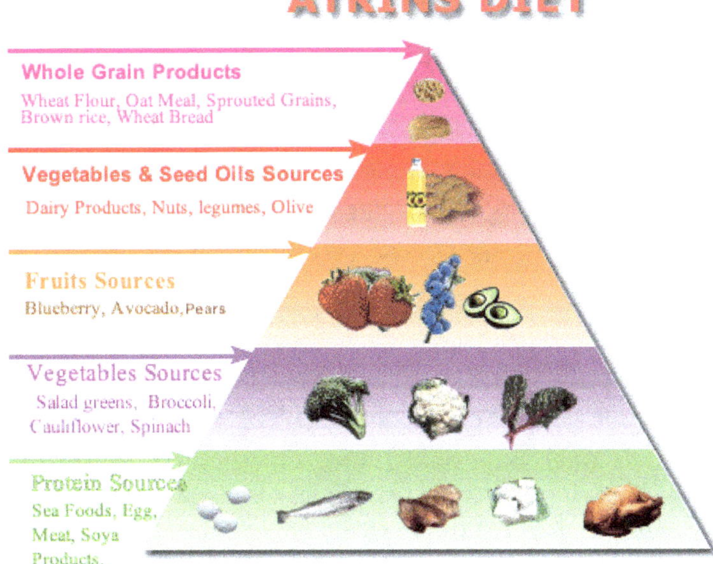

Other benefits: Numerous studies show that low-carb diets, like the Atkins diet, may reduce many risk factors for disease, including blood triglycerides, cholesterol, blood sugar, insulin, and blood pressure.

Compared to other weight loss diets, low-carb diets also better improve blood sugar, "good" HDL cholesterol, triglycerides, and other health markers.

The drawback: As do other very low-carb diets, the Atkins diet is safe and healthy for most people but may cause problems in rare cases.

6. The Zone Diet

The Zone Diet is a *low-glycemic load* diet that has you limit carbs to 35–45% of daily calories and protein and fat to 30% each. It recommends eating only carbs with a low glycemic index (GI) (Already discussed GI). The GI of a food is an estimate of how much it raises your blood glucose levels after consumption. The Zone Diet was initially developed to reduce diet-induced inflammation, cause weight loss, and reduce your risk of chronic diseases.

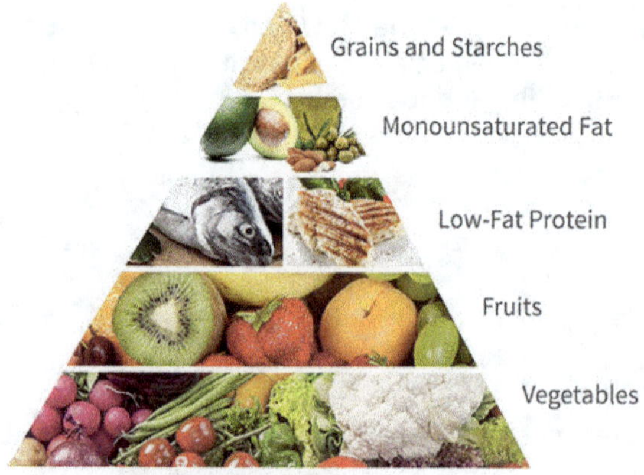

Zone Food Pyramid

How it works: The Zone Diet recommends balancing each meal with 1/3 protein, 2/3 colorful fruits and veggies, and a dash of fat — namely monounsaturated oil, such as olive oil, avocado, or almonds. It also limits high-GI carbs, such as bananas, rice, and potatoes.

Weight loss: Studies on low-GI diets are rather inconsistent. While some say that the diet promotes weight loss and reduces appetite, others show very little weight loss compared to other diets.

Other benefits: The greatest benefit of this diet is a reduction in risk factors for heart disease, such as reduced cholesterol and triglycerides.

One study suggests that the Zone Diet may improve blood sugar control, reduce waist circumference, and lower chronic inflammation in overweight or obese individuals with type 2 diabetes.

The drawback: One of the few drawbacks of this diet is that it limits the consumption of some healthy carb sources, such as bananas and potatoes.

8. Intermittent Fasting

Intermittent fasting cycles your body between periods of *fasting and eating*. Rather than restricting the foods you eat, it controls when you eat them. Thus, it can be seen as more of an eating pattern than a diet.

The most popular ways to do intermittent fasting are:

- **The eat-stop-eat method:** Involves *24-hour fasts once or twice per week* on non-consecutive days.

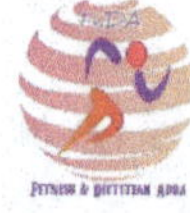

68

- **The 5:2 diet:** On two non-consecutive days of the week, you restrict your intake to 500–600 calories. You do not restrict intake on the five remaining days.
- **The 16/8 method:** Involves skipping breakfast and restricting your daily eating period to eight hours, subsequently fasting for the remaining 16 hours of the day.

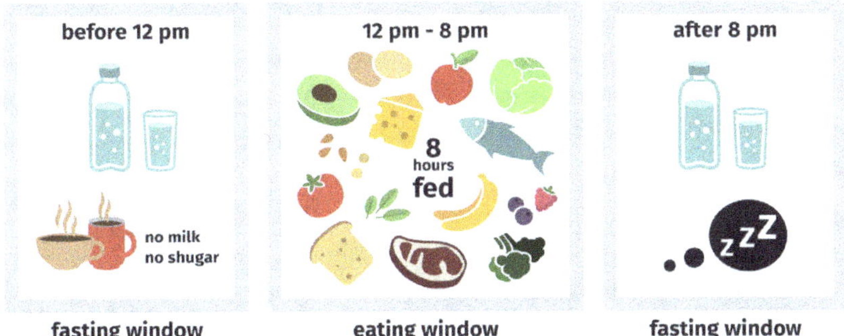

- **The Warrior Diet:** Eat small amounts of raw fruits and vegetables during the day and one huge meal at night.

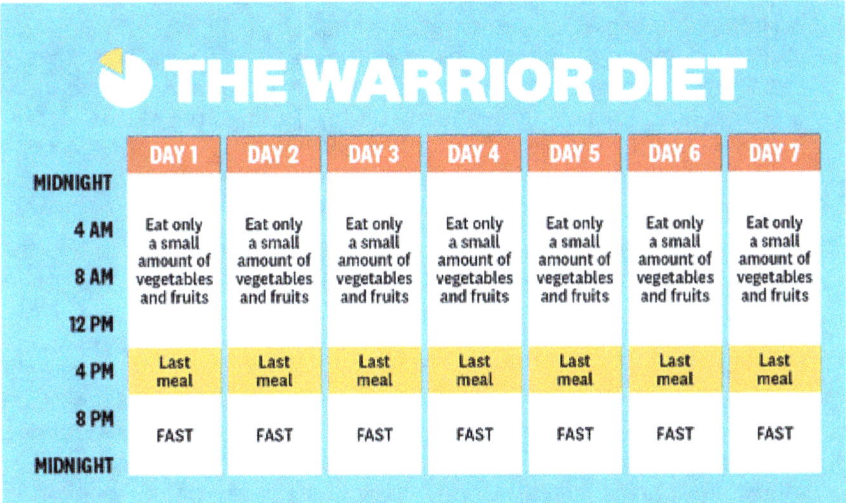

THE WARRIOR DIET

	DAY 1	DAY 2	DAY 3	DAY 4	DAY 5	DAY 6	DAY 7
MIDNIGHT / 4 AM / 8 AM / 12 PM	Eat only a small amount of vegetables and fruits	Eat only a small amount of vegetables and fruits	Eat only a small amount of vegetables and fruits	Eat only a small amount of vegetables and fruits	Eat only a small amount of vegetables and fruits	Eat only a small amount of vegetables and fruits	Eat only a small amount of vegetables and fruits
4 PM	Last meal	Last meal	Last meal	Last meal	Last meal	Last meal	Last meal
8 PM / MIDNIGHT	FAST	FAST	FAST	FAST	FAST	FAST	FAST

How it works: Intermittent fasting is commonly used for weight loss because it leads to relatively easy calorie restriction.

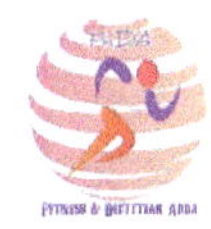

It can make you eat fewer calories overall — as long as you don't overcompensate by eating much more during the eating periods.

Weight loss: Intermittent fasting is generally very successful for weight loss. It has been shown to cause weight loss of 3–8% over a period of 3–24 weeks, which is a lot compared to most weight loss diets.

In addition to causing less muscle loss than standard calorie restriction, it may increase your metabolic rate by 3.6–14% in the short term.

Other benefits: Intermittent fasting may reduce markers of inflammation, cholesterol levels, blood triglycerides, and blood sugar levels.

Furthermore, intermittent fasting has been linked to increased levels of human growth hormone (HGH), improved insulin sensitivity, improved cellular repair, and altered gene expressions.

Animal studies also suggest that it may help new brain cells grow, lengthen lifespan, and protect against Alzheimer's disease and cancer.

The drawback: Although intermittent fasting is safe for well-nourished and healthy people, it does not suit everyone. Some studies note that it's not as beneficial for women as it is for men.

In addition, some people should avoid fasting, including those sensitive to drops in blood sugar levels, pregnant women, breastfeeding moms, teenagers, children, and people who are malnourished, underweight, or nutrient deficient.

9. KETO Diet

Scientists have shown that when either lean or obese individuals exercise after eating a high fat meal, their fats are broken down and oxidized in skeletal muscle, making them healthier. These results show for the first time how a high fat diet and exercise stimulate the breakdown of fats and may help design ways to reduce excessive fat in the body.

Ketosis is a metabolic process. When the body does not have enough glucose for energy, it burns stored fats instead. This results in a buildup of acids called ketones within the body. (vast description in chapter 11)

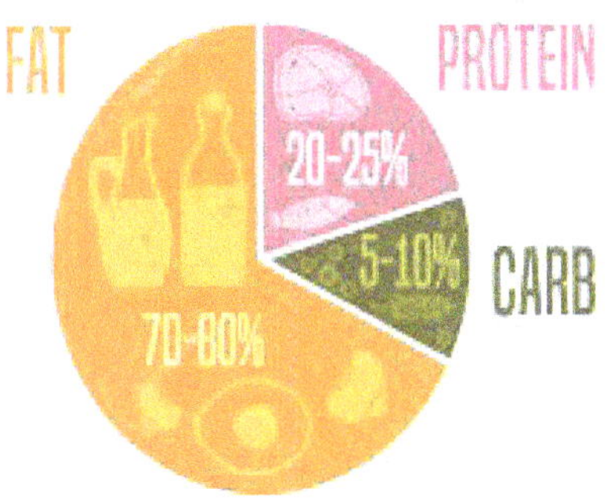

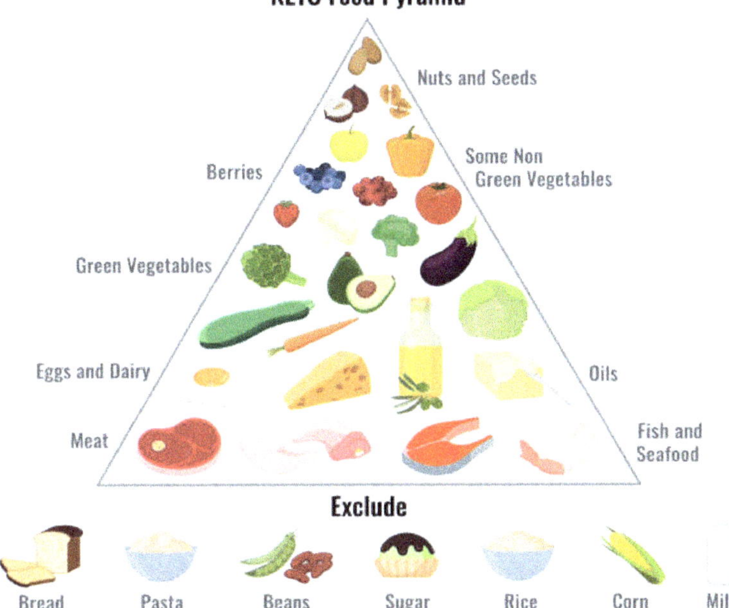

WHAT ABOUT DIETARY CHOLESTEROL?

Cholesterol is not fat. It is a waxy substance found only in foods of animal origin: meat, poultry, seafood, egg yolks and dairy products. Humans do not need to consume any cholesterol because our cells can produce all the cholesterol our bodies need for use in cell membranes and hormones. High intakes of dietary cholesterol can raise LDL cholesterol and can increase heart disease risk in other ways.

However, this effect is generally not as strong as that of saturated fats and trans fats. People who have high blood cholesterol levels, heart disease or diabetes should limit their intake of dietary cholesterol. The foods listed below are relatively high in dietary cholesterol:

Dietary Cholesterol

- Egg yolks or whole eggs: limit to 2 per week
- Organ meats: liver, brains, kidney and sweetbreads
- Shrimp and squid/calamari (one serving a week is okay)
- Meat, poultry and seafood in large amounts (i.e. more than 5 or 6 oz./day)

HERE ARE SOME GENERAL GUIDELINES FOR HEALTHY EATING

- The most important rule of healthy eating is not skipping any meal. Skipping meals lowers your metabolic rate. Normal eating includes 3 major meals and 2 snacks between meals. Also, Never skip breakfast. It is the foremost vital meal of the day.
- Learn simple ways to prepare food. Healthy eating doesn't have to mean complicated eating. Keep meal preparation easy, eat more raw foods such as salads, fruits and vegetable juices, and focus on the pleasure of eating healthy food rather than the calories.
- It is important to stop when you feel full. This will help you maintain your weight to an extent. This also will help you remain alert and feeling your best.
- Drink lots of water. Keep a bottle of water near you while working, watching TV, etc.
- Variety of foods should be used in the menu. No single food has all the nutrients.
- To improve the cereal and pulse protein quality, a minimum **ratio of cereal protein to pulse protein should be 4:1**. In terms of the **grains, it will be eight parts of cereals and one part of pulses**.
- Eat five portions of fruit and vegetables every day.
- Keep a supply of healthy snacks to hand. This will stop you from eating an unhealthy snack when hungry.
- Remove all visible fat from food before you cook it – take the skin off chicken and trim the white fat off any meat.
- Limit stimulants such as caffeine, alcohol and refined sugar.
- Limit the number of times you eat out to once a week. Take your own packed lunch to work.

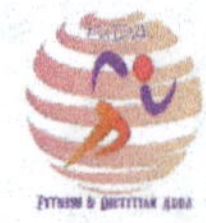

- Only eat things you like the taste of – find what works for you and don't force yourself to eat things just because they're good for you.

HEALTHY COOKING TIPS

With today's fast life, cooking a meal in the traditional style is extinct. People mostly opt for eating less healthy fast foods, ready to eat meal packets, etc.

To make a healthy meal, the most important thing is to cook it at your home, rather than opting for outside cooked food. Explore healthy ways to add variety to your meals as repetition can cause boredom. Infuse your diet with the excitement and good taste you crave for.

Here are a few suggestions for cooking healthily. Having to choose healthy food does not mean you need to give up on your favorites. Think of how you can turn your favorites into a healthy option. For instance:

- Decrease the meat and add more vegetables to your dishes.
- Use whole wheat flour instead of refined flour when you bake.
- Blot your fried foods to take off the extra oil.
- Use low-fat yogurt instead of mayonnaise
- Add cut fruits to your curd, rather than having flavored yogurt
- Try to skim milk instead of a normal one.
- Use non-stick cookware to reduce the need for oil to cook.
- Microwave or steam your vegetables rather than boiling to avoid loss of nutrients.
- Fats in your foods should be maintained to a minimum.
- Choose lean meats and skim dairy products. Fats are good in the form of nuts, seeds, fish, olives when they are accompanied by other nutrients. Some amount of fats while cooking is good as it helps the body to absorb fat-soluble vitamins.
- If you wish to use oil, try cooking sprays or apply oil with a pastry brush. Cook in liquids (such as vegetable stock, lemon juice, fruit juice, vinegar or water) instead of oil. Use low-fat yogurt, low-fat soymilk evaporated skim milk or cornstarch as a thickener instead of cream.
- Choose to scrub the vegetables than peel as there are many nutrients in the skin. When you have to boil the vegetables, retain the vitamin-rich water and use it as a stock in another preparation.
- Switch to a reduced salt wholemeal or wholegrain bread.

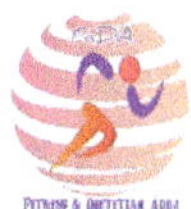

- For sandwiches, limit your use of spreads high in saturated fat like butter and cream cheese; replace with scraps of spread or alternative nut spreads or low-fat cheese spreads or avocado. Choose reduced-fat ingredients like low-fat cheese or salad dressing.
- Add a lot of vegetables to your sandwich to make it healthier.

Appetite and Hunger

Appetite is **a person's desire to eat food**. It is distinct from hunger, which is the body's biological response to a lack of food. A person can have an appetite even if their body is not showing signs of hunger, and *vice versa*.

Hunger occurs when the body recognizes that it needs more food and sends a signal to the brain to eat.

Food poisoning

Food poisoning, also called *foodborne illness*, is **illness caused by eating contaminated food**. Infectious organisms — including bacteria, viruses and parasites — or their toxins are the most common causes of food poisoning.

Symptoms:
- Nausea
- Vomiting
- Watery or bloody diarrhea
- Abdominal pain and cramps
- Fever

___________________By_Mr._Hitesh_Andel___________________

74

Chapter 9: Diet Planning Tool

Diet Planning

A healthy diet consists of vegetables, fruits, and whole grains. It *may include lean meats, poultry, fish, beans, eggs, and nuts.* And it's low in saturated fats, trans fats, cholesterol, salt, and added sugars.

Principles of diet planning

The diet-planning principles :

1. Adequacy : Maintaining adequate levels of energy, nutrients, movement and rest for optimal health.
2. Balance : Balancing different food groups, and consuming foods in the right proportion.
3. Calorie (energy) control : Consuming the appropriate number of calories to maintain a healthy weight depending on your. metabolism and exercise levels.
4. Nutrient density : Focussing on creating a diet that is nutrient dense without being high in calories.
5. Moderation : Learning how to be moderate with foods that are higher in fat or sugar.
6. Variety : Exploring a varied diet that provides all the nutrients necessary for good health.

Meal planning

Meal planning is the act of thinking ahead about what you'll make for meals and snacks and getting prepared. You'll eat healthier meals and snacks. Meal planning gives you the opportunity to think about what you like to eat and how those foods help nourish your body.

Diet planning Vs. Meal Planning

- ☐ Diet means what we eat the entire day or week or month, while Meal is what we eat in a single sitting. It may be our Breakfast, Lunch, Snacks or Dinner.

- ☐ Diet planning involves the entire meals of the day or week or month.

- ☐ Meal planning involves the act of planning out portions of meals for the entire week or month.

- ☐ Diet is a wider term while Meal is a part of Diet.

- ☐ **Meal** = one specific thing we eat (lunch is a meal, dinner is a meal and chips is a meal etc)

- ☐ **Diet** = Refers to everything we regularly eat.

Classification of Diet plan

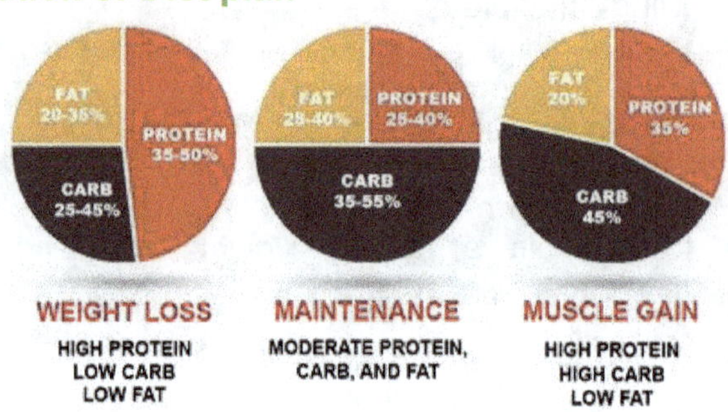

Total Calorie

Total Calorie consist of the following :
- ☐ BMR
- ☐ NEAT
- ☐ DIT
- ☐ Exercise Activity Thermogenesis

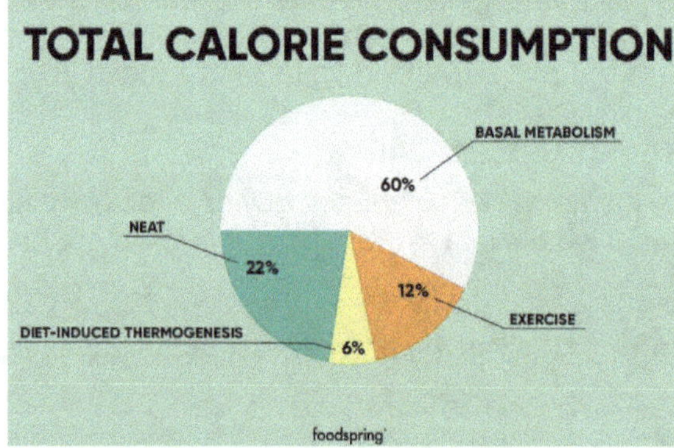

Total daily energy expenditure (TDEE), that is the number of calories you burn each day.

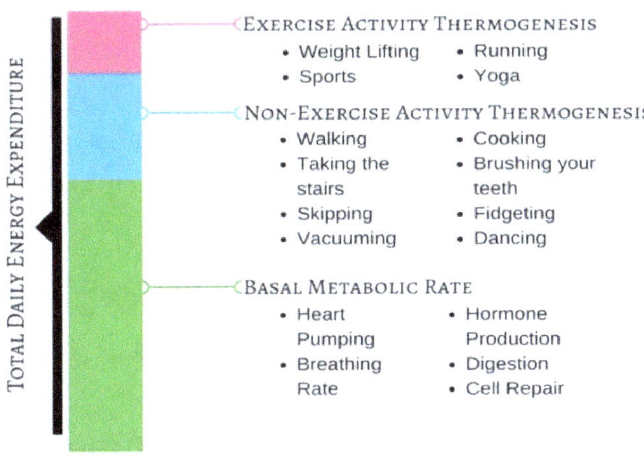

Basal Metabolic Rate (BMR) : (Option 1)

The basal metabolic rate (BMR) is the *rate of energy expenditure of a person at rest*; it eliminates the variable effect of physical activity. The BMR accounts for approximately 60% of the daily energy expenditure.

BMR is **just the number of calories your body burns at rest** and does not account for the calories you need to walk, talk, exercise, etc. When thinking about your caloric needs for a meal plan, you must account for your current activity level or your increased activity level if you plan to exercise more.

BMR Formula
(Harris-Benedict)

MEN

BMR = 66.47 +
(6.24 × weight in lbs)
+ (12.7 × height in inches)
− (6.755 × age)

WOMEN

BMR = 655.1 +
(4.35 × weight in lbs)
+ (4.7 × height in inches)
− (4.7 × age)

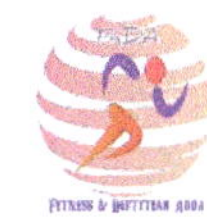

77

BMR FORMULAS

$$BMR = \begin{array}{l}(10 \times \text{weight [kg]}) \\ + (6.25 \times \text{height [cm]}) \\ - (5 \times \text{age [yrs]}) + 5\end{array}$$

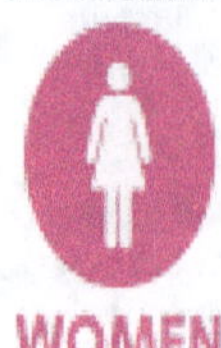

$$BMR = \begin{array}{l}(10 \times \text{weight [kg]}) \\ + (6.25 \times \text{height [cm]}) \\ - (5 \times \text{age [yrs]}) - 161\end{array}$$

Calorie-Calculation Harris Benedict Formula

Once you've calculated your BMR, this is then put into the Harris Benedict Formula , which calculates your total calorie intake required to maintain your current weight. This is as follows:

- For sedentary (little or no exercise)
    = BMR x 1.2
- For lightly active (light exercise/sports 1-3 days/ week)
    = BMR x 1.375
- For moderately active (moderate exercise/sports 3-5days/week)
    = BMR x 1.55
- For very active (hard exercise/sports 6-7 days a week)
    = BMR x 1.725

Let's have an example;

I'm 29 years 5'10" Hight (178cm) and my weight is 68.6 Kgs (151 lbs.).

= (10 x weight in Kg) + (6.25 x height in cm) - (5 x age in year) + 5
= (10 x 68.6) + (6.25 x 178) - (5 x 29) + 5
= (686) + (1112.5) - (145) + 5
=1658.5 BMR Kcal.
Now applying Harris Benedict Formula on above outcome, I'm considering myself lightly active, So
= 1658.5 x 1.375 **= 2280**

Non-exercise activity thermogenesis (NEAT)

Non-exercise activity thermogenesis (NEAT) is the energy expended for everything we do that is not sleeping, eating or sports-like exercise. It ranges from the energy expended walking to work, typing, performing yard work, undertaking agricultural tasks and fidgeting.

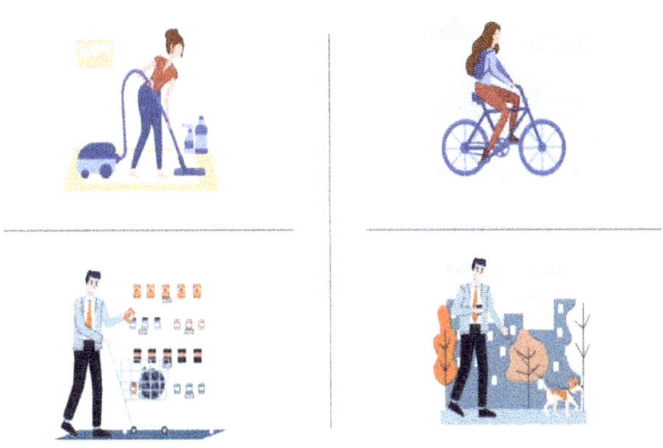

Diet-Induced Thermogenesis (DIT)

Diet-Induced Thermogenesis (DIT) is the production of heat that occurs after eating - which contributes to the body's resting metabolic rate. DIT is also called the thermic effect of food. It activates sympathetic nervous system activity and increases Resting Metabolic Rate.

Exercise Activity Thermogenesis

Exercise activity thermogenesis is energy expended from exercise that we intentionally engage in (anything you do at the gym, going on a brisk run, etc.). We focus on activity thermogenesis – calories burned while exercising – when attempting to lose weight.

Lean Mass calculation

`Now we all know how to calculate our BMR, but it is to be noted that before calculating the BMR we should know the value of our body fat. Basically our body fat percentage decides if we need to calculate your BMR by considering our total body weight or our lean body mass. Lean Body Mass is basically the fat free mass in our body. It's also not your muscle mass so kindly don't get confused between the two. Normally if your body's fat percentage is more than 20 (in case of men)/28 (incase of women), it is advised to consider the

lean mass to calculate the BMR. There is a very simple formula that is been used to calculate the lean mass:
i.e.: **Lean Mass = Total Body Weight – (Body Fat % x Total Body Weight).**

For example, if a person is weighing 100 kgs and has body fat % of 40 then his lean mass would be 100 – (0.40 x 100) = 60kgs. So the above person should calculate the BMR by putting his lean mass i.e. 60kgs instead of total body weight i.e. 100kgs.

Maintenance calories: (Option 2)

Maintenance calories are precisely **the number of calories your body needs to support energy expenditure**.

To determine the appropriate amount of calories to consume for our planned gaining or cutting phases, we must first *establish a baseline target* that would theoretically result in no change.

"The estimation of caloric intake that would simply keep you at your current body weight is referred to as your maintenance calories."

To determine maintenance, you can either track body weight and calories to ascertain the relationship between the two variables, or you can estimate maintenance calories with an equation. Both ways give you a value for maintenance calories.

To calculate your maintenance calories, it's essential to know your TDEE (total daily energy expenditure). This number includes *three main components:*

- BMR (basal metabolic rate)
- NEAT (non-exercise activity thermogenesis)
- Exercise

Estimating Maintenance by Calculation

Now keeping in mind that there are huge amounts of individual variation here, a good way to *ballpark* this for most people would be to first take your *body weight in pounds and multiply it by 10 (or multiply your body weight in kilograms by 22) and then multiply that value by an activity multiplier.*

Here I continue my previous example, let's do a calculation, weighs 151lb (68.6 kg), when we multiply by 10 (22) we get a theoretical baseline of 1509 calories.

Step 1: Baseline Multiplier; Not Accounting for Any Activity
68.6 x 22 = 1509 calories

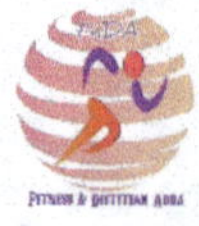

Then we multiply that by an activity multiplier. This also includes something called **NEAT**, which stands for *non-exercise activity thermogenesis*. Or more simply put, any activity outside of exercise, including subconscious movement.

Step 2: Using An Activity Multiplier

Using An Activity Multiplier	
LIFESTYLE & TRAINING FREQUENCY	ACTIVITY MULTIPLIER
Sedentary plus 3-6 days of weight lifting	1.3 – 1.6
Lightly active plus 3-6 days of weight lifting	1.5 – 1.8
Active plus 3-6 days of weight lifting	1.7 – 2.0
Very active plus 3-6 days of weight lifting	1.9 – 2.2

Baseline Multiplier x Activity Multiplier = Estimated Calories For Body weight Maintenance

Depending on lifestyle and individual differences, these calculations can equate to a 1962 – 3320 calorie range for maintenance in our 151lb (68.6 kg) example.
Again I'm considering myself Lightly Active, so
= 1509 x 105
=2263 Kcal (~2280 as calculated in BMR through Harris Benedict Formula)

"How do I know which value to choose, what determines each level of activity?" However, if you want to get started faster, just *take the middle value of 1.7 as your multiplier.* Then, if you gain or lose weight too quickly after 2–3 weeks, just adjust your intake. This is a perfectly valid approach.

The Difference Between BMR And Maintenance Calories

Many people wrongly assume that the BMR = maintenance calories. That is not so. BMR (basal metabolic rate) is the amount of calories that your body needs just to function. That means to sustain all the vital organs like the heart and the basic functions like breathing.

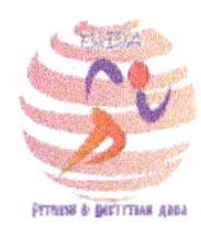

81

Most people, besides breathing and staying at rest, also do other things during the day, like walking and sometimes even being active.

All these activities require a greater expenditure of calories than the BMR. So in order to change your weight you need to find what your MAINTENANCE calories are.

Maintenance calories are your BMR calories + the amount of calories that you expend throughout the day on going around doing your daily activities (for example walking or doing sports).

If your goal is to gain weight, then you should eat more calories than your maintenance calories. For people that are trying to lose weight, they should first calculate their BMR and their maintenance calories. After that they need to eat less calories than their maintenance calories, but still more than their BMR.

Body Mass Index (BMI)

Using body mass index (BMI) is one way a person can determine whether or not their weight is healthy for them. **BMI takes both height and weight into consideration.**

Body Mass Index (BMI) is a person's weight in kilograms divided by the square of height in meters. A high BMI can indicate high body fatness.

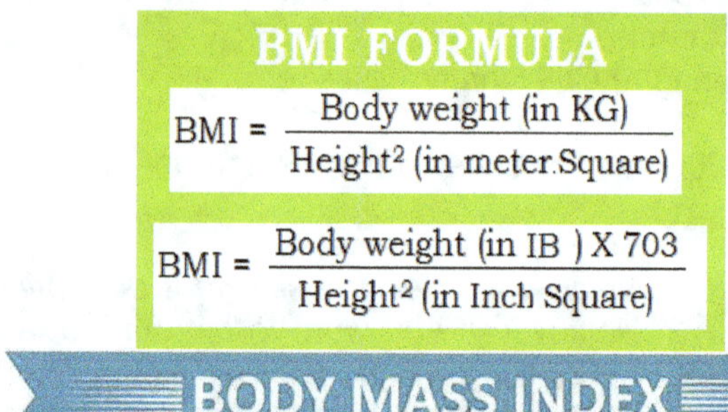

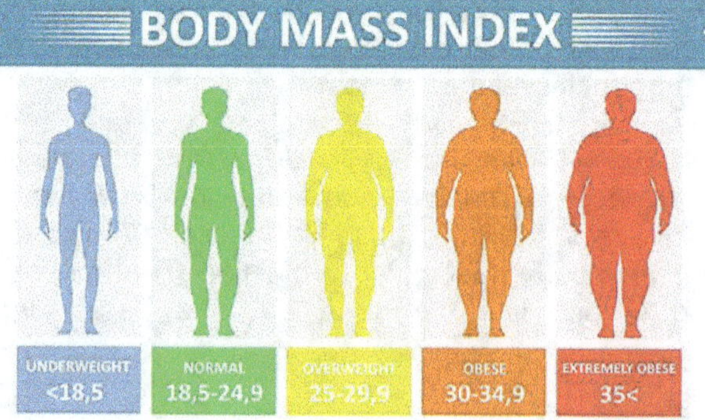

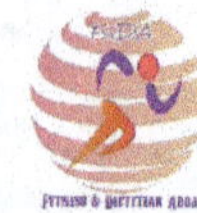

82

Metabolism

The process in which our body uses fuel to provide energy to our body is called Metabolism. Food contains ingredients which our body can use as fuel. But even this fuel is not yet in the form of an energy that can be used immediately.

If I give you a fully charged battery, try using it to bake an egg. Possible? No. Having an energy containing fuel does not mean that it is ready to use. It all starts with food, and its

Metabolically Active Ingredients -
Fat, Fiber, Long Carbohydrates, Short Carbohydrates (Sugar in other words), Protein
1g of Fat = 9 Calories
1g of Carbohydrates = 4 Calories
1g of Fiber = 2 Calories, they are extremely important in making digested food leave your body.
1g of Protein = 4 Calories
1g of Alcohol = 7 Calories

Our body can extract at least the following three kinds of fuel from what we ingest:
1. Free Fatty Acids
2. Glucose
3. Amino Acids
4. Fat → Free Fatty Acids
5. Fibers (used for excreting ingredients)
6. Long carbohydrates → Shorter → Glucose
7. Shorter carbohydrates ('sugars') → Glucose
8. Proteins → Amino Acids
Now that we know what the actual fuels are, it's time to understand how they are stored in the body. Different kinds of fuels are stored in different forms and different amounts, and in different locations.

Understanding Metabolism

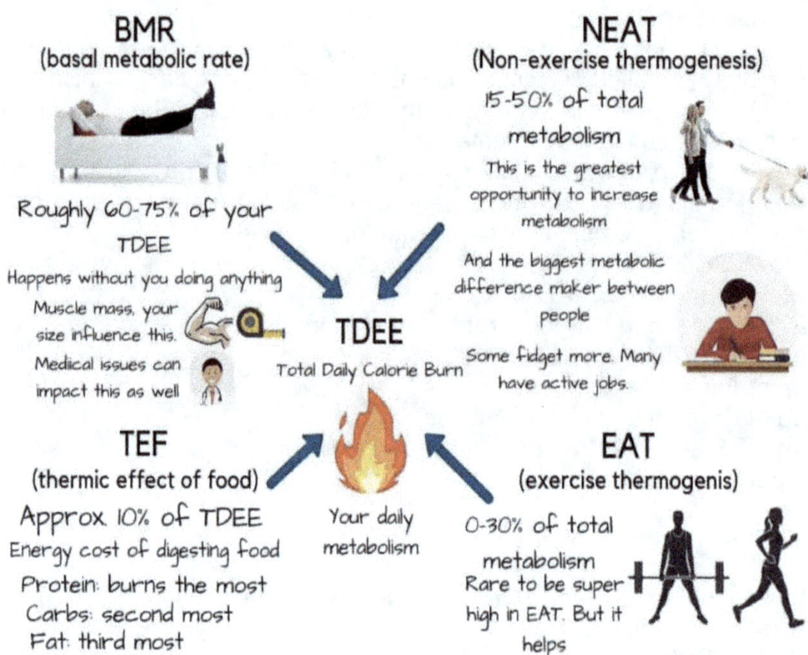

1. FATTY ACIDS: Almost any cell can store fatty acids, they can also be transported directly in the bloodstream - no conversion is needed. If it turns out that you do not have enough cells to store all fatty acids, your body can easily generate special 'adipocytes' (fat cells), which together, form the so-called 'adipose tissue'.

As can easily be observed, the body easily stores tens of kilos of fat. As each kilo of fat can power an individual for many days, an average person actually carries enough energy in the form of fat to survive for a month. An overweight person often carries enough fuel to survive for many months.

But All this doesn't make fat bad. Just remember, you can survive without carbs, but without essential fats, your brain will simply stop working. So never ever cut down fat completely from your diet. You need essential fats every single day for your survival.

2. GLUCOSE: Glucose is a very small molecule and easily travels from cell to cell. This makes it easily transportable. This mobility is not very well suited for actually storing sugars, so for storage, sugars are converted to glycogen. Glycogen is a molecule which consists of

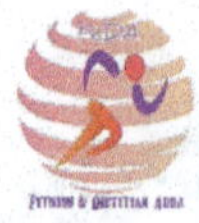

84

smaller glucoses. This size and aggregation makes it easier to store glucose.

As glycogen, sugar is stored in the liver and in muscles. Both liver and muscles can convert glucose to glycogen. The liver can convert glycogen back to glucose but muscles cannot. Muscles can however use glycogen directly if needed, or release it into the bloodstream.

What is very notable, is the limited amount of sugars which can be actually stored. Ingested glucose and small carbohydrates like table sugar travel nearly directly to the bloodstream. While this allows the body to rapidly utilize ingested sugar, what this eventually means is that the amount of glucose allowable in blood can be easily exceeded.

People of average weight will generally have in the order of 5 grams of glucose in their blood at any specific time. Levels above 10 grams are considered too high.

This means that a regular candybar, which contains approximately 30 grams of sugar, actually poses a great challenge to the body.

When glucose arrives (via the food we eat) in excess of 10 grams, the body releases insulin, which instructs the liver and muscles to absorb glucose from the blood. Furthermore, all parts of your body which can run on glucose start doing so as well.

Consequently, the burning of fatty acids for energy production is reduced. Beyond the bloodstream, the body can store a few hundred grams of glucose. Amounts differ with the actual body mass and the physical condition of each individual body, but are generally in the order of approximately 150 grams. The glucose storage can generally be depleted in a single day, making it a very short-term fuel.

Complex carbohydrates cannot be transferred directly to the bloodstream and must be converted first, which can take quite some time. That is actually a good thing, because this delay ensures that the blood isn't overflooded with glucose.

3. PROTEINS AND AMINO ACIDS : These are found throughout the body, either bunched up as proteins or freely available amino acids. They are the building blocks and can be used to form muscle fibers, or cells, or lots of other things, all of which can also be broken down again into proteins or even amino acids. It is a reversible process.

Proteins are broken down into amino acids in the intestine and then brought to the liver, where they are partly reassembled and partly released into the bloodstream.

Compared to glucose, a lot of protein is available for use at any one time. The blood alone will contain in the order of approximately 100 grams.

Compared to either glucose or fatty acids, amino acids also have "huge" uses. It can also be stated that you ARE a big aggregation of amino acids. They make up your DNA and mostly everything else that is interesting in your body.

Almost everything can be converted to everything else in the body. But not always and not everywhere. Important conversions are:

(A) From Glucose to Glycogen to Stored Fat

As mentioned earlier, this is done when your sugar intake has exceeded the storage capacity. This happens a lot.

(B) From Stored Fat to Glucose

Creating glucose from non-glucose parts is called Gluconeogenesis and this is very important. It helps power the brain using long-term energy storage (fat).

Role of water

Let's start with discussing blood. The blood serves as a medium for taking fuel to the cells, but it also works to transport away stuff the cells have discarded. What this means is, if left uncleansed of these waste products, the bloodstream would quickly become polluted. So, there are at least three organs working on cleaning it up: the two kidneys and the liver.

The Kidneys function primarily as sophisticated filters. As long as things are kept wet enough, they are able to remove waste from the blood by osmosis. This waste may be further treated, and is eventually sent to the bladder for excretion out of the body.

The Liver is a much more complex organ capable of advanced-level functions. It actually converts a lot of waste products into usable substances again. It can also break down molecules which cannot be filtered by the kidneys. Almost all energy conversions taking place in your body are centered around the liver.

The kidneys primarily need water to function - they need to be wetter than your blood. If they cease to be so, they become unable to filter the waste-laden blood, leaving (part of) this job to the liver. The liver then becomes occupied doing that and has less time or capacity left for conversions. When this occurs, the body may actually enter a

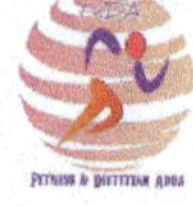

'starvation' state. The liver is unable to furnish the brain with sugar and no other energy sources are available. This quickly leads to dizzy spells and general incompetence.

Effectively, what this indicates is the overwhelming importance of staying hydrated. Water is a brilliant blessing to our body, although most of us seldom realize its
importance. Staying hydrated has tremendous health benefits, not just for your skin, or your metabolism, or your digestion, but for optimal functioning of vital body processes.

_____________________By_Mr._Hitesh_Andel________________

Chapter 10: Diet Plans

Introduction

When we have understood all the necessary terms and calculations for making a diet, we move towards the diet plans. Here in this chapter we will see the basic diet plans as per requirements of lean gaining, losing or maintaining the weight.

These are the Nutrients must be consisted in a good Diet for Adult :

1. Carbohydrates and Fibers : 45 to 65% of total calorie
2. Fat : 25-35% of total calorie
3. Protein : 0.8 to 2 gm of per KG body weight
4. Vitamins and Minerals : Trace

1.   How many carbs we need

On average, people should get 45 to 55% of their calories from carbohydrates every day. On the Nutrition Facts labels, the Daily Value for total carbohydrates is 275 g per day. This is based on a 2,000-calorie daily diet. Your Daily Value may be higher or lower depending on your calorie needs and health.

2.   How does Fat affect us

Around 25-35% of the total energy you take in should come from fat. For example, for a 2000 kcal diet, the recommended amount of fat you should take in is 55g-65g. Taking in more fat than needed will lead to a build-up of extra calories. If you keep on taking in more calories than you burn through physical activity, you will gain weight and increase your chance of being overweight. The additional fat in your body can increase your risk of getting diabetes, heart disease, high blood pressure and some forms of cancer.

3.   How many protein we need

A safe level of protein ranges from 0.8 grams of protein per kilogram of body weight [2.2 lbs.], up to 2 grams of protein per kilogram for very active athletes.

Calculation of macros

As you already know 1g Carbs contain 4 Kcal, 1g Protein contains 4 Kcal and 1g of Fat Contains 9 Kcal.

Lets have an example of a **2000 kcal** Diet for an average person weighted 60 kgs.

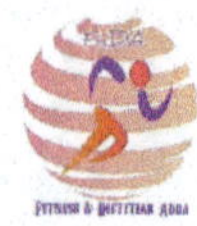

Protein :

Person who works out in the gym should consume 0.8 to 2g of protein per kg of body weight.
I.e. 60 x 0.8 (min considering) = **48g of protein**
1 g protein has 4 Kcal
So 48 g protein shall have 48 x 4 = 192 Kcal

Fat :

Fat must be consumed in the portion of 25-35% of total calorie. So here I am taking the lower side just for understanding.
Total Kcal 2000 X 25% = 500 Kcal
1 g Fat has 9 Kcal
So 500 Kcal would be equal to **56g of Fat**.
500 Kcal / 9g = 56g

Carbs :

Now the remaining calories will be compensated by the Carbs.
2000 - 192 - 500 = 1308 Kcal
1g Carb has 4 Kcal
So 1308 Kcal / 4g = **327 g Carbs.**

Conclusively, I can say the following is to be considered while preparing above 2000 Kcal Diet:

Carbs   :   327g (carbs including fibers)
Protein   :   48g
Fat   :   56g

Adding some fruits and vegetables for Vitamins, Minerals and Fibers.
Consuming 8 to 10 glasses of water.

There are various types of Diet as per requirements:

LOW CARB DIET (25:35:40)

This would be required to trim excess body fat, while making slow lean gains. It is effective, however it takes a lot of time to show results (ideal for anyone who's new).

ZONE DIET (40:30:30)

This is the diet that has higher amounts of carbohydrates. This is ideal for the ones who absolutely love carbohydrates. This is also perfect

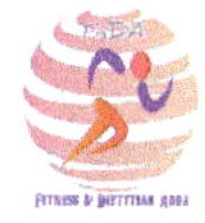

for the people who have high tolerance towards carbohydrates which is commonly seen among the people with high muscle mass.

DEPLETION DIET (DYNAMIC)

To reduce body fat% dramatically and bring definition to your muscles in a very short period (not for people with body fat above10%). This diet focuses mainly towards glycogen depletion and also reduces the subcutaneous water retention to a certain degree.

WARNING: Depletion diet requires immense knowledge and understanding about body composition and should only be attempted if you're an advanced level athlete and are below 10% body fat. It can screw up your metabolism if done wrong, not to mention causing muscle loss and hormonal imbalance.

KETOGENIC DIET (5:35:60)

A ketogenic diet will also target your body fat levels and like the depletion diet, it will also reduce your water retention to a large extent. It engages your body in producing more ketones hence the name, Keto diet. It is an ideal diet to start with if your goal is fat loss but would be sub-optimal for muscle gain.

Before you start planning your diet, you have to calculate your BMR as mentioned in the previous Chapter. Figure out how many calories you're going to consume to reach your target goal and then based on the diet, you have to divide your macronutrients into ratios.

Low Carb Diet

Since we're looking to get shredded by a low carb diet, our **Fat:Carbs:Protein Ratio** should be low in carbs and balanced protein and fats depending on the rest of our intake. A **40:25:35 F:C:P ratio** is decent for this in most cases.

Of course there will be slight variation, but that is fine. It's just to give you an idea and stress on the fact that your carb intake will be lower while fat intake will be the highest (keeping protein constant).

How does it help? Fats help in satiety. And this diet will help you to stay satiated, with enough fiber of course. Also, it's good for anyone who's insulin resistant or diabetic (more on this later. *Do not experiment on your own if you are diabetic*. I suggest an expert to handle such cases).

To help you understand more efficiently, let me give you an example :

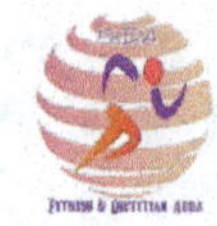

I am 29-year-old and 5'10 weighing 68.6 KG. After calculating my BMR (say 1658.5) I calculate my daily calorie needs using the Harris Benedict equation(Described in previous Chapter) and my calorie intake comes to about 2280 calories a day considering I do light exercise (just an example).

Now to start losing weight (fat, not muscles) I will design my diet in such a way that I will have a macro ratio of 40:25:35 (F:C:P) in a calorie deficit mode.

How many calories do you need to reduce? It's up to you. However, the body does not like dramatic changes and it retaliates in a dramatic manner, leading to loose skin, water retention etc. (will address these problems in later part). It's better to lose weight gradually than dramatically. So I'd suggest a cut of 200-300 calories in the first couple of weeks to start noticing change. And then further down by 400-500 in subsequent weeks to start fat loss and turn the body into a fat burning machine. You should never reduce more than 1000 calories, as it would most probably slow down your metabolism.

Protein has 4, Carb has 4 and Fat has 9 calories per gram. So if I were to receive 2280 kcals in a day, I would use the macro ratio of 40:25:35 to calculate my macro in grams.

I calculated using the above formula. I get the following: 143gm carbs, 200gm protein and 101gm of fat.

Now it is tough to find food which has only protein or carbs or fat alone. Most of the foods have a mix of all. In this case you can look at the labels or *use Google* and a little bit of brain to find out what combination will give you the above ratio.

You can use the following table to choose your staples.

PROTEIN	CARBS	FATS	FIBER
Chicken	Green Vegetables	Paneer	Vegetables
Eggs	Fruits	Yogurt	Sprouts
Fish	Rice	Cheese	Fruits
Whey Protein	Legumes	Olive Oil	
Tofu	Sprouts	Flaxseed	
White Mushrooms	Banana	Fish Oil	
Paneer/Cheese	Wheat	Nuts	
Soybeans/chunks	Quinoa	Coconut	

This limited list is only for your reference (in no particular order). There are several others you can choose from.

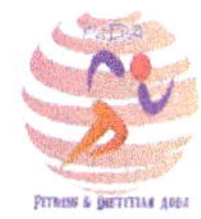

91

Zone Diet

Simply change the macro ratio in the above diet to **40:30:30** and it becomes a **Zone Diet** for *lean muscle gains* if you stay on a *small surplus.* However, if you keep the total calories on a deficit, it will help you drop your body weight.

You can introduce more carbs like oats, brown rice, sweet potato etc. It is always a good idea to consume carbs around the workout period. Also, I suggest you have carbs around 1 to 2 hours before the workout.

What really matters is the intake and your expenditure though. The macro ratio is simply for better adherence. Choose whatever suits you. And what really helps you to lose fat would be your resistance training. So make sure you don't skip your training.

Depletion Diet

You will need **iron will and** a **rock solid determination** to complete two weeks of this diet. I would not suggest extending it beyond that period for multiple reasons including but not limited to hormonal damage, poor metabolism, and regaining weight. So if you do it, do it 100% right or do not do it at all. It's called a Depletion Diet because you will deplete your body of carbohydrates and sugars, which will leave you with fat as the only available option in the body compelling it to make the "Switch" thereby allowing body to use fat as its primary fuel (of course, coupled with the right resistance training and proper protein intake).

Once again, I am not going to give you a magic formula. The idea here is to teach you, to help you understand how things work so that you can design your own diet. Now let's set a few things straight.

Your body including your muscle tissues is 70% water. Your muscles are not as big as you think they are. They appear big at any point of time as they are holding a lot of glycogen and water in them.

Generally, 100 gm of your lean muscle tissue will hold up to 2 gm of glycogen, and each of this 2gm of glycogen will further associate itself with around 3 grams of water. So if a person has 30kg of lean muscle tissue, i.e. 30,000gm of muscle tissue, the muscles will store up to 600gm of glycogen which will further store 600x3= 1800gm of water. That's 1.8 kg of water.

People who start with a depleted diet often get confused when they see their weight dropping initially. It is this water glycogen weight that shows a massive drop initially. Even though there is no fat loss, you can lose up to 2 to 5 kg of your bodyweight at the beginning

92

of the diet depending on your lean muscle tissue and water storage capacity.

Feeling a bit disappointed...? You shouldn't be! It is actually not a bad thing. If you are into a contest prep, you will realize how this water and glycogen manipulation can make you stand out in the crowd (Has to do with bodybuilding. Others can ignore).

Well, let's get deeper. So now you know that proper fat loss is not really an easy game and to start seeing any results, you will have to get your basics right. And that is the main idea behind any diet, be it Atkins diet, or low carb diet.

One way of doing that would be to gradually reduce the caloric intake. But returning to a depleted diet, the goal would be to gradually reduce the carb intake every week or few days, so that eventually our intake is less than 20 gm per day, and simultaneously, we'll be supplementing with enough protein to make sure muscle loss is minimum. And don't worry if your muscles appear flat, it's because your muscles are getting rid of the excess glycogen and water. They will fill out once you're back to your normal routine.

Also, the initial few days of carb depletion will be very challenging as your body will struggle to adjust with lower energy supplies. Remember at this point it will be reluctant to use fat as an energy source.

However once your glycogen levels are completely depleted, you will experience what is called "the switch" i.e. your body will start using fat and you will feel a *tremendous surge* in your energy levels. This should happen typically during the second week. The key is to keep pushing through the first week.

The following is a sample depletion diet which I use. This is what I personally use, if you compare this with my normal diet (previously discussed), you will notice that I have eliminated all sources of carbs here except spinach (since we need dietary fiber at all times and the carb content in vegetables can be ignored).

I agree that this is neither an ideal diet, nor is it properly balanced. But then, I'm sharing it only to give you a rough idea. Now that you know the concept I am sure you can come up with a diet which looks perfect for you. You can even add other vegetables and protein sources in it.

AROUND 8AM
1 Scoop Protein Shake
1 Tbsp Flaxseed
4 Egg White Omelette

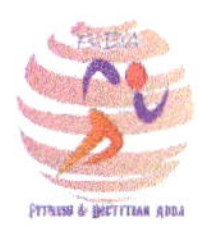

93

AROUND 12PM
8 Egg White Scramble
1 Bowl Spinach (200gm)

AROUND 4PM
4 Egg Whites

POST WORKOUT
2 Scoops Protein

AROUND 8PM
8 Scrambled Eggs
1 Bowl Spinach 200gm

AROUND 10PM
1 Scoop Protein(depends)

AROUND 11Pm
Sleep

NOTE : During the first week you can have brown rice as a measure of your carbs and you can gradually keep reducing it. E.g, 100 gm, then 80, then 60 and so on and during the conditioning week, no brown rice.

Please note that you will have to **drink more water than usual**. Since your muscles will lose glycogen and consequently water, you will continuously need to drink water to replenish and keep them hydrated.

Peak Week and Contest Preparation

This is just for your information. Remember when I said that during the initial period of carb depletion, your body only loses water weight. And how that is not a bad thing. Now I'll explain how.

See once your muscles are depleted of glycogen and water, they have a tendency to store more glycogen. If during normal state your muscles stored 2gm of glycogen per 100gm of lean muscle tissue, after depletion it can store up to 4gm of glycogen and hence more water. Bodybuilders and athletes take advantage of this situation.

Following a depletion diet, they start carb loading, which lets them appear fuller and huge on stage and all the carb will get used up to fill increased glycogen levels. Also a lot of subcutaneous (under the skin) water will be pulled into the muscles giving a dry and ripped

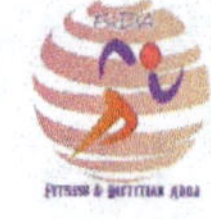

94

look. However, this only works for people who are below a body fat% of 10 or less, as it won't make a difference if you have more fat mass.

Agreed, it's the calories at the end of the day that matters when it comes to weight loss or weight gain, but choosing to ignore the right source because you read some new research or an article by some of the leading names in the industry may actually not be beneficial for your ultimate goals. You will get results, Will the results be optimal? Far from it actually.

So people professing that eating Dal Chawal, mixing carbs and fats, and eating sweets is allowed because it is within their TDEE. Here's something that might burst your bubble:

Not all calories are treated in the same way by the body, for eg. Both fructose and glucose yield 4 calories per gm, but they are very different when it comes to being metabolized by the body.

Fats have a different metabolic pathway so do amino acids, and mind you all this is conditional, based on different circumstances, the usage in the body can change.

One such example is the *ghrelin* levels. *Ghrelin* is your *hunger hormone*. When it is up, it makes you feel hungry. Different foods have different effects on ghrelin levels, whole foods containing fructose or glucose will trigger more ghrelin levels and will make you eat more compared to proteins or fats. This is one more reason why it is easy to stick to a low carb diet compared to a high carb diet at the same calories.

Different foods can impact your metabolism negatively or positively, be on an ice-cream diet for 1600 calories for a few days and you'll see your metabolism will drop and even at 1600 calories you will find it difficult to lose weight. Try the same with a high protein or a high fat diet and you'll be losing weight pretty sharply. Same calories and different results, anyone doubting the results can try it on themselves if they dare.

A gram of omega-3 fatty acid will provide the same amount of calories as a gram of omega-6 fatty acids, yet one is good while the other is not that much good for health. (Will share in next edition).
So you see a calorie is not just a calorie, and anyone who says that at the end of the day that calories are calories and source doesn't matter, does not know what they are talking about.
Sources of calories matter! Be wise, while picking the sources.

PEAK WEEK TECHNIQUE
MONDAY
CARBS- 50% DROP

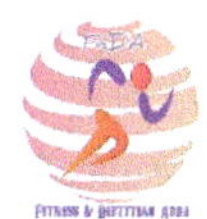

WATER- 6 LTR
SALT- NORMAL

TUESDAY
CARBS- FURTHER 50% DROP
WATER- 6-7 LTR
SALT- NORMAL

WEDNESDAY
CARBS- FURTHER 50% DROP
WATER- 6-7 LTR
SALT- 50% DROP
PROTEIN & FATS GOES UP BY 5-10%

THURSDAY
CARBS- ZERO
WATER- 6-7 LTR
SALT- FURTHER 50% DROP
PROTEIN & FATS GOES UP BY 5-10%

FRIDAY
CARBS= MONDAY
WATER- 3 LTR
SALT- MINIMUM

SATURDAY
CARBS- 2* MONDAY
WATER- 1 LTR
SALT- ZERO (ONLY INTRODUCE 2-3 HOURS PRIOR TO SHOOT)

Reverse Dieting

The single most relevant factor that is responsible for a 'no-more' fat loss zone or fat loss plateau is the downregulation/slowdown of your metabolism. This is because as you cut down calories, no matter how small the deficit is, metabolism will start to come down. Simply because the body will try to preserve energy for survival. In this process our body will reduce the production of metabolism friendly hormones like *thyroid*, *free testosterone* and *leptin* to maintain energy balance. Not just that, but your body will downregulate a lot of its operations.

Reverse Dieting Protocol:

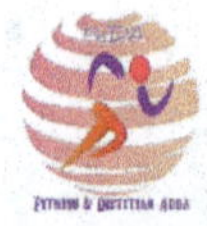

Now you might claim that decreasing calories result in weight loss, so adding up calories will result in weight gain. This is where maintenance calories have to be kept in mind while reverse dieting specifically for weight loss.

A slight increase in weight while reverse dieting does not necessarily mean that you are adding fat. That will not happen unless you go beyond your maintenance calories or overlook macro distribution. This slight increase in weight will be intracellular water retention or gain in muscle glycogen.

For example, if you are on a calorie deficit diet for weight loss, you start off by preparing a diet chart with calories equal to your BMR, suppose your BMR = 1600 calories and you are following a low carb diet so you would start with calculating your macros for 1600 calories i.e. 25:45:30 – C/P/F. This would come up to 80gms carbs, 160 gms proteins and 71 gms fat.

Now after following a chart with the mentioned macros for a week, you should increase the calories by 100-150 gms (depends upon the week's results) so for the next week you will have to modify your diet chart and make a new chart for 1600 + 100 = 1700 calories, similarly the macros would change to 85gms carbs, 170gms proteins and 75gms fat.

Every week we keep increasing the calories by 100-150 based on the improvement and keep repeating the procedure till our fat loss stalls. The stage at which this happens, this stalling, this stage indicates that the person has reached his/her maintenance calories and thus they should ideally go back to their BMR value and repeat the whole thing again.

DIETING STRATEGY – Everyone wants to get muscles, but you have to decide for yourself. Do you want to look like a freak show or aesthetically built? If the answer is latter, then you should follow this guideline

- If you can see your abs, you can start by adding around 150-200kcals to your maintenance calories with a low carb diet initially for 4 weeks and then continue on a zone diet for as long as you want.
- If you can't see your abs but are already fit, then switch to low carb till you are shredded enough and then stick to a zone diet for as long as you want.

Whichever diet you choose for dropping your fats or for gaining muscles, you need to maintain a caloric deficit or a caloric surplus respectively.

Do not keep reducing calories - most people, if they don't get results, keep on reducing calories further and further, which is not good. What you are actually doing is you are harming your metabolism. This is true for most people who tend to lose weight by doing a starvation or crash diet. And they gain the weight back again very soon.

If you do the above mentioned diets correctly, you will see that your metabolism will only get better, you may even keep losing weight despite higher calorie intake.

However, you should be regularly lifting heavy weights as well. Your training should be on point. Not only during the dieting down phase, but always.

While preparing Diet this guideline must be followed :

- Eat a wide variety of foods from the **five** food groups:
    - Plenty of colourful vegetables, legumes/beans
    - Fruit
    - Grain (cereal) foods – mostly wholegrain and high fibre varieties
    - Lean meats and poultry, fish, eggs, tofu, nuts and seeds
    - Milk, yoghurt, cheese or their alternatives, mostly reduced fat. (Reduced fat milks are not suitable for children under the age of two years.)
    - Drink plenty of water.

- Limit foods high in **saturated fat**, such as biscuits, cakes, pastries, pies, processed meats, commercial burgers, pizza, fried foods, potato chips, crisps and other savoury snacks.

- Replace high fat foods containing mostly **saturated fat** with foods containing mostly polyunsaturated and monounsaturated fats. Swap butter, cream, cooking margarine, coconut and palm oil with unsaturated fats from oils, spreads, nut butters and pastes, and avocado.

- Limit foods and drinks containing added **salt**, and don't add salt to foods in cooking or at the table.

- Limit foods and drinks containing added **sugars**, such as confectionery, sugar-sweetened soft drinks and cordials, fruit drinks, vitamin waters, energy and sports drinks.

- Limit alcohol. Drink no more than two standard drinks on any day to reduce your risk of harm from alcohol-related disease or injury over your lifetime, and drink no more than four standard drinks on any occasion. For women who are pregnant or thinking about getting pregnant, or breastfeeding, not drinking alcohol is the safest option.

Together with following the healthy eating guidelines, aim for at least 30 minutes of moderate intensity physical activity, such as walking, every day.

Benefits of above mentioned five foods :

Fruit, vegetables and legumes all provide vitamins, minerals, dietary fibre and nutrients. Most are low in calories and can help you to feel full longer.

Eating lots of colourful choices from this food group will give your body different nutrients. It can also protect against chronic diseases including heart disease, stroke, diabetes and some cancers.

Vegetables – How much to put on your plate *each day* :

- Younger children – 2.5 serves for 2–3 year olds and 4.5 serves for 4–8 year olds

- Older children – 5 to 5.5 serves for older children and adolescents

- Adults and pregnant women – 5–6 serves

- Breastfeeding mums – 7+ serves.

- *A standard serving is about 75 grams* (100–350 kilojoules); for example, ½ cup cooked green or orange vegetables (such as broccoli or carrots) or 1 cup green leafy or raw salad vegetables.

- **Fruit** – How much to put on your plate each day :

- Younger children – 1 serve for 2–3 year olds and 1.5 serves for 4–8 year olds

- Older children, adolescents and adults, including pregnant and breastfeeding women – at least 2 serves.

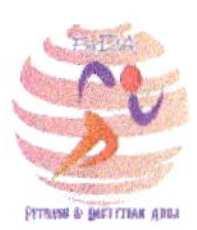

- ***A standard serve is 150 grams*** (350 kilojoules); for example, a medium apple or banana, or two kiwifruits or plums. Try to eat whole fruit and not fruit juice.

Legumes are also made up of protein, so they're a useful substitute for meat. Choose from split peas, kidney beans, baked beans (navy beans), soybeans, chickpeas, lupin, and lentils, among others.

Legumes/beans (as a source of protein) – How much to put on your plate each day :

- Children – 1 to 2.5 serves, depending on age

- Men – 2.5 to 3 serves, depending on age

- Women – 2 to 2.5 serves, depending on age

- Pregnant women – 3.5 serves

- Breastfeeding women – 2.5 serves

- **A standard serving is 500–600 kilojoules**; for example, 1 cup of cooked or canned lentils, chickpeas or split peas, or 170 grams of tofu.

Wholemeal or **whole grain** foods, such as wholemeal and wholegrain bread, brown rice, quinoa and oats, are better for you than refined grain (cereal) foods because they provide more dietary fibre, vitamins and minerals. Whole grains may protect against heart disease, type 2 diabetes, excessive weight gain, and some cancers.
    Grain (cereal) foods that are high in saturated fats, added sugars and added salt, like cakes, muffins, pies, pastries and biscuits, are 'extras' or 'sometimes foods' in this food group.

Grain foods – How much to put on your plate each day:

- Younger children – 4 serves

- Older children and adolescents – 7 serves

- Women – 3 serves for those over the age of 70; 6 serves for women less than 50 years of age; 8.5 serves for pregnant and breastfeeding women

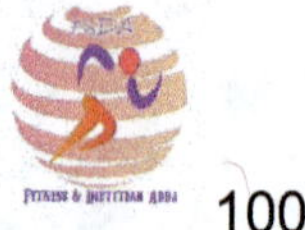

100

- Men – 4.5 serves for those over the age of 70 years; 6 serves for younger men.

- A standard serve is 500 kilojoules; for example, one slice of bread or ½ cup cooked porridge. At least two-thirds of choices should be wholegrain varieties.

Lean meats, poultry, fish, eggs, tofu, nuts and seeds, and legumes/beans are all rich sources of protein. Eating a variety of these foods each day will provide the protein you need, as well as a range of other nutrients, including iodine, iron, zinc, vitamins (especially B12), and essential fatty acids.

The Dietary Guidelines recommend that you eat one to three serves of food from this group each day, depending on your age. If you are pregnant, three to four servings a day are recommended.

Lean meats, poultry, fish, eggs, tofu, nuts and seeds, legumes/beans – How much to put on your plate each day

- Children – 1 to 2.5 serves, depending on age

- Men – 2.5 to 3 serves, depending on age

- Women – 2 to 2.5 serves, depending on age

- Pregnant women – 3.5 serves

- Breastfeeding women – 2.5 serves

- A standard serve is 500–600 kilojoules; for example, 80 g cooked lean poultry (100 g raw), 100 g cooked fish fillet (about 115 g raw), 65 g cooked lean red meat (about 90 – 100 g raw), two large eggs (60 g each), 170 g tofu, 30 g nuts or seeds, or 150 g cooked legumes.

Milk, yoghurt and cheese are rich sources of calcium and other minerals, protein, and vitamins. They can protect against heart disease and stroke, and reduce the risk of high blood pressure, some cancers, and type 2 diabetes. Dairy is also good for bone health. Choose varieties low in saturated fat and added sugar.

If you prefer to avoid dairy, go for alternatives with added calcium, such as calcium-enriched soy or rice drinks. Make sure they contain at least 100 milligrams of calcium per 100 millilitres.

Milk, yoghurt and cheese or alternatives – How much to put on your plate each day

- Children – 1.5 to 3.5 serves, depending on age

- Men – 2.5 to 3.5 serves, depending on age

- Women – 2.5 to 4 serves, depending on age

- Pregnant women – 2.5 serves

- Breastfeeding women – 2.5 serves

- **A standard serving is 500–600 kilojoules**; for example, a cup of milk or ¾ cup yoghurt.

'Extras' or 'sometimes foods'

Some foods are known as 'discretionary foods', 'extras' or 'sometimes foods' because they should only be consumed sometimes – they're not a regular part of a healthy diet.

Extras are higher in kilojoules, added sugar, saturated fat, and added salt, such as commercial burgers, pizza, alcohol, lollies, cakes and biscuits, fried foods, and fruit juices and cordials.

Timing your food intake

When you eat also plays a part in a healthy diet. The biggest food timing tip is to eat breakfast.

Breakfast literally means 'to break the fast' from your last meal at night to your first meal of the following day.

Breakfast skippers are more likely to be tempted by unhealthy choices later in the day and to eat bigger servings at their next meal. Children who skip breakfast generally have poorer nutrition and poorer performance at school.

Other food timing tips are:

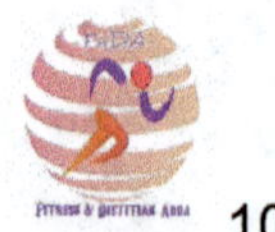

102

- Eat regularly: Eating regular meals at set times helps you to get all the servings from the five food groups. Aim for breakfast, lunch and dinner, and two snacks.

- Listen to your body: Follow your body's hunger and satiety signals (eat when you're hungry and stop when – or before – you're full).

- Stop to eat: Take your time when you dine, and turn off the TV or computer. Notice your food, and your body's signals.

- Avoid eating dinner late at night: This gives your body time to digest and use the energy from your meal. Try a small glass of milk or a cup of decaffeinated or herbal tea if you need a late-night snack.

- Eat larger at lunch and smaller at dinner: The body digests best at peak energy times, which occur from around noon until 3 pm. If you can't handle a bigger lunch, try splitting it into two smaller meals and eating one at noon and the other mid-afternoon. Eating dinner an hour earlier also aids evening digestion.

- Eat about 45 minutes after exercise: This will reduce the amount of energy being stored as fat because the body will use it to replenish low glycogen stores.

Carbohydrates and glycaemic index

Carbohydrates are the body's preferred energy source. They are found in many foods, such as breads, breakfast cereal, rice, pasta, noodles, fruit, potato and starchy vegetables, corn, dried beans and lentils, sugar, milk and yoghurt. Eating a carb at every meal fuels the body throughout the day.

Include a variety of good-quality carbs, such as fresh, canned or dried fruit; rice, bread, quinoa and pasta (preferably whole grain or high fibre varieties); and legumes in your healthy diet.

Carbohydrate-containing foods are rated on a scale called the glycaemic index (GI). This rating (between zero and 100) is related to how quickly their carbohydrate content is digested and absorbed into the bloodstream, and the effect it has on blood glucose levels .

Low GI foods (GI less than 55) absorb into the bloodstream slowly and give sustained energy throughout the day. *Examples*

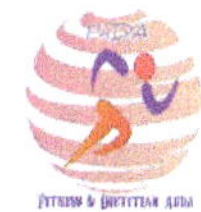

103

include whole grain bread, pasta, oats, apples, apricots, oranges, yoghurt, milk, dried beans and lentils.

High GI foods (55 or more on the GI scale) are **quickly** digested and absorbed into the bloodstream. *Examples of high GI foods are white and wholemeal bread, processed cereals, short grain rice, potatoes, crackers, watermelon.*

It's ok to include both high and low GI foods in your diet, but tending towards the lower end of the GI scale in your food choices is shown to improve health.

Here's a quick look at the glycemic index of some common foods we eat across India:

Food groups	Low GI (0-55)	Medium GI (55-69)	High GI (> 70)
Cereals	Barley, oat bran, quinoa, daliya	Whole wheat, rye, muesli, basmati or brown rice	White rice or bread, puffed rice, beaten rice (poha), refined flour (maida), instant oats, cornflakes, cake, and cookies
Pulses	Green gram, black-eye peas (lobia), soybean, chickpea (chhole), kidney bean (rajma)		
Vegetable	Leafy greens (such as spinach, fenugreek, amaranth), brinjal, green beans, cauliflower, carrot, cucumber, tomato, broccoli	Peas, yam, sweet potato	Pumpkin, white potato
Fruits	Apricots, apple, grapefruit, oranges, kiwi, peaches and pears, plum, berries	Papaya, banana, cantaloupe, mango, figs, pineapple, dried fruits and raisins	Watermelon, dates
Milk and Milk Products	Milk and milk products such as curd, buttermilk	Ice-cream	

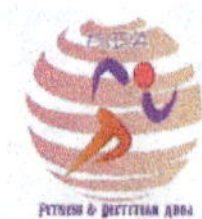

Others	Vegetable soup, peanuts, flax seeds, almonds, walnuts, pumpkin or sunflower seeds, seafood, eggs, meat, spices	Soft drinks, honey	Energy drink, pizza, fast foods, sugar, jaggery, chocolates

Satiety Index

It's an excellent tool when choosing the right foods for your weight loss food program. It tells you to minimize your hunger pangs, making it easier to follow your weight loss intentions. The Satiety Index-tool ranks different foods on their ability to satisfy hunger.

The index is based on a study performed at the University of Sydney, Australia in which they compared the filling effects of different foods. It's clear that certain foods satisfy hunger much better than others. The test was done by giving a group of volunteers portions of 240 calories from different food sources and then measuring how much they ate when they were allowed to eat again after two hours.

The index of white bread was set at 100. Foods scoring higher than 100 are more filling than white bread and those under 100 are less filling.

The index only takes into consideration how long a certain food will keep you full, it doesn't say anything about nutritional value or calorie content.

Best "non-hunger" foods

Protein is the nutritive substance that satisfies hunger best based on its energy content and ability to make you feel full over the longest period of time.

Carbohydrates are also good if you exclude plain sugar and well known fast carbs (white
bread, etc.).

Fatty foods are surprisingly not filling, even though people expected them to be. Good news for dieters.

Foods rich in fiber also rank high and contain few calories.

Generally speaking, foods that rank high and satisfy your hunger for a longer period of time are foods with high protein, -water- and/or fiber content. These foods will help make you feel full, literally by filling your stomach, and with a full stomach you can more easily avoid nibbling.

How To Use The Satiety Index

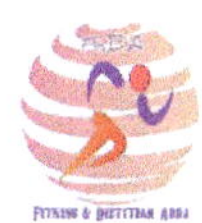

105

As with any index that measures just one thing, the satiety index has to be put into a context, it can't be used on its own.

Let's look at some examples:
Plain boiled potatoes showed to be the most satisfying food tested according to energy content, three times more satisfying than white bread.

A lot of people, having learned about the Glycemic Index, avoid potatoes during a diet as it doesn't have a low glycemic index but a medium one. From a nutritional point of view plain boiled potatoes are an excellent choice of diet food, full of vitamins and fibers. Potatoes don't make you gain weight, as long as you don't eat them with butter, sour cream, cheese etc. So maybe it's time to reevaluate the potato because of its brilliant ability to satisfy hunger? As your stomach shrinks, you can remove it from your diet if you want to.

Another example:
Pop corn ranks high and it also contains a greater amount of bulk for each calorie. You can eat a lot of popcorn without consuming a lot of calories (assuming you're eating them without oil or butter!) when you want to snack, like in front of the television or while reading a book. The best thing, of course, is to not snack at all but if you feel you just have to have something, the value of popcorn as a weight loss food should not be underestimated, it is so much better than potato chips.

Final outcome of The Satiety Index

So, a good diet for weight loss should, from the satiety point of view, contain at least some slowly-digested carbs and protein.

Together with what you already know of calorie content it's easy to choose the right food. Good choices are lean meat and chicken without the skin, food rich in fiber, like beans and lentils and whole meal bread.

Also preferable are foods rich in water. Vegetables are especially great for weight loss; they contain lots of nutritional value, few calories and they are filling.

The Satiety Index has, as does the glycemic index, limitations. It doesn't tell you anything about the nutritional value of the food; only how well a certain food satisfies your hunger.

If you look at the list you will see that jelly beans score high. One of the reasons, according to the researchers, is that jelly beans made the test volunteers slightly nauseous and therefore they didn't

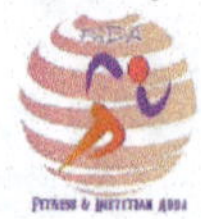

106

feel like eating for quite a while after eating their portion of 240 calories of jelly beans. Jellybeans are also high in sugar, making them a bad choice from the perspective
of the glycemic index.

As you see, the Satiety Index is one of many tools you can use together with your knowledge of nutrition to make your weight loss easier.

The Satiety Index List			
All of the following foods are compared to white bread, ranked as "100".			
Bakery Products	**Rank**	**The list with the most filling food at the top**	
Croissant	47%	Potatoes, boiled	323%
Cake	65%	Ling fish	225%
Doughnuts	68%	Porridge/Oatmeal	209%
Cookies	120%	Oranges	202%
Crackers	127%	Apples	197%
Snacks and Confectionary		Brown pasta	188%
Mars candy bar	70%	Beef	176%
Peanuts	84%	Baked beans	168%
Yogurt	88%	Grapes	162%
Crisps	91%	Whole meal bread	157%
Ice cream	96%	Grain bread	154%
Jellybeans	118%	Popcorn	154%
Popcorn	154%	Eggs	150%
All-Bran	151%		

Porridge/Oatmeal	209%	**Cheese**	146%
Breakfast Cereals with Milk		**White rice**	138%
Muesli	100%	**Lentils**	133%
Sustain	112%	**Brown Rice**	132%
Special K	116%	**Honey Smacks**	132%
Cornflakes	118%	**All-Bran**	151%
Honeysmacks	132%	**Crackers**	127%
Carbohydrate-Rich Foods		**Cookies**	120%
White bread	100%	**White pasta**	119%
French fries	116%	**Bananas**	118%
White pasta	119%	**Jellybeans**	118%
Brown Rice	132%	**Cornflakes**	118%
White rice	138%	**Special K**	116%
Grain bread	154%	**French fries**	116%
Whole meal bread	157%	**Sustain**	112%
Brown pasta	188%	**White bread**	100%
Potatoes, boiled	323%	**Muesli**	100%
Protein-Rich Foods		**Ice cream**	96%
Lentils	133%	**Crisps**	91%
Cheese	146%	**Yogurt**	88%

Eggs	150%	Peanuts	84%
Baked beans	168%	Mars candy bar	70%
Beef	176%	Doughnuts	68%
Ling fish	225%	Cake	65%
Fruits		Croissant	47%
Bananas	118%	Table adapted from S.H.A. Holt, J.C. Brand Miller, P. Petocz,and E. Farmakalidis,	
Grapes	162%	A Satiety Index of Common Foods, Table adapted from S.H.A. Holt,	
Apples	197%	European Journal of Clinical Nutrition, September 1995, pages 675-690.	
Oranges	202%		

According to some authors, ingestion of high glycemic index diets tends to enhance appetite and promote positive energy balance. Short-term investigations have generally demonstrated that ingestion of low glycemic index foods results in greater satiety and lower energy intake than high glycemic index foods.

The importance of the post-workout snack

During exercise, the muscles use up stored glucose, called glycogen, and levels become depleted. Endurance sports, such as running, use up more glycogen than resistance activities, such as weightlifting. Another effect of exercise is that the muscles develop small tears.

Getting the right nutritional balance after exercise restores energy levels and reduces fatigue, helping the body to repair muscles and build strength for future workouts.

Proteins, carbohydrates, and healthful fats are all essential for the body's recovery.

Protein

Exercise supports muscle growth, but the body can only build upon existing muscles if they recover after each workout.

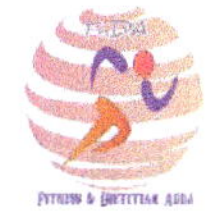

109

Consuming protein after exercise helps the muscles to heal and prevents the loss of lean mass. Lean mass contributes to a muscular and toned appearance.

Carbohydrates

Carbohydrates are macronutrients that help the body to recharge and restore its fuel supply.

Anyone who exercises more than seven times a week should consume plenty of carbohydrates, as they quickly replenish glycogen levels.

What about fat?

Many people believe that consuming fat after exercising slows digestion and the absorption of nutrients. For some types of fat, this may be true.

However, there is little information about the post-workout effects of fat calories. It may be a good idea to limit fat intake after exercise, but low levels of fat are unlikely to inhibit recovery.

Meal Frequency

This simply refers to how many times you consume nutrients in a day. That might be the old-school recommendation of seven to eight meals per day from an IFBB professional bodybuilder, or that might be two to three meals per day in a certain window from someone in the intermittent fasting crowd. Generally, I'd say we should end up somewhere in the middle of those two extremes.

Now there is a decent amount of research on pretty much everything from one meal a day all the way up to 14 meals per day, and surprisingly limited investigation of the more moderate frequencies of four to five meals per day. But collectively, the data suggests if you are eating in the range of a relatively normal number of meals, say three to six, this doesn't make a huge difference as far as the actual outcome of body composition. What we can say though is that some blips on the radar start to come up when you get on the extreme ends of very low or very high meal frequencies.

When you start touching the low end (two meals or less) or the high end (more than six meals a day), you can potentially start running into issues with adherence. Less than three meals and you tend to go long periods of time without food and that can affect your hunger and ability to maintain consistency.

You'll also eat very large meals that can sometimes cause you to develop unhealthy relationships with food where you train yourself to consume an enormous amount of calories at each sitting.

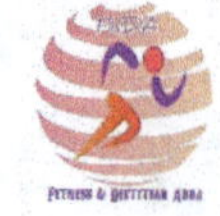

110

Likewise, you can run into the opposite problem eating more than six meals a day. Having tiny meals every hour or two that don't satisfy you can leave you constantly focused on food. Either end of the spectrum can exacerbate hunger control.

So, my conservative recommendation that combines practical experience, theory, and the limited studies we have, is to consume somewhere between three to six meals per day in most cases.

But that said, if you have previously found success with slightly more or fewer meals than this, that's not necessarily a bad thing.

If you do fine on two meals per day or seven meals per day, feel free to stick with it. There are plenty of competitive bodybuilders who have found a great deal of success following very high meal frequencies (six to eight meals per day), and likewise there are many folks who have followed an intermittent fasting approach to eating who have had personal or competitive success eating two meals per day (usually involving skipping breakfast) with only whey protein or BCAA prior to training - buy the whey save yourself some money and just use protein powder instead of BCAA if you decide to train 'fasted'.

In fact, when variations in meal frequency from two to seven meals per day are studied, no significant differences in energy expenditure are found. However, inconsistent meal timing across the week, as opposed to maintaining a consistent meal frequency, can decrease energy expenditure (to a small degree)and insulin sensitivity. So, if you are satiated by your current meal frequency setup, it is not socially stressful or inconvenient, and it works for you, don't think you have to change it.

Really, it's just a good idea to have a consistent structure to your diet. Regular meal times, and habits (like having a protein serving, a fruit serving, and a veg serving at each meal) can go a long way towards consistency, adherence, reducing decision fatigue, and getting results.

Finally, for those of you who are larger individuals in a gaining phase with a high caloric intake, you might have trouble consuming the high number of calories that you need with a more moderate meal frequency. In your case, it might be better for you to aim for six or even seven meals daily. Hunger is not going to be an issue that needs to be controlled. If anything, being too full can become an issue, so if you need to increase meal frequency to reduce meal size so you can get 5000 calories, go for it.

Should I Gain or Should I Cut?

The answer to this question depends on more than just your current body composition. It's not quite as simple as saying: cut if you are high in body fat, gain if you are not. There is also an interaction with training experience. Indeed, I wouldn't advise someone with obesity who is just starting a weight training program to purposely go on a fat loss plan. Just becoming more active alone can give someone who was previously sedentary more finely tuned hunger signals, and body-fat percentage will go down even if muscle is gained without fat mass losses. Also, metabolic health will improve purely from resistance training without dieting.

In this case, I'd only advise you to institute a caloric deficit once the initial "magic" of newbie gains ends, and if at that point you still had a goal of lowering your body fat (which as I said, may happen anyway just from lifting regularly).

In the case of someone who is generally not very muscular, but is also higher in body fat than average (often referred to as "skinny fat"; I'm not a fan of the term, but it hopefully helps you understand what I'm referring to), I also don't recommend cutting.

The times the answer to this question are cut and dry, is when you aren't a novice. If you have a few years under your belt of training, and you fit into the "intermediate" or "advanced" categories, gaining or cutting does pretty much just come down to your body fat level.

However, the answer to this question is also not as critically important as you might believe. There is a common notion that if you aren't reasonably lean, efforts at gaining will produce a disproportionate amount of fat and little in the way of muscle. This concept is called your 'P-ratio', which is simply defined as the proportion of fat to muscle you put on when gaining weight.

Indeed, there is research showing that very lean people — who are naturally lean, not who dieted — gain more lean body mass during periods of overfeeding, and people with obesity gain more body fat during periods of overfeeding.

However, what two things that are frequently misunderstood are:

1) putting on more lean body mass when overfeeding occurs in naturally lean people who walk around lean. If you dieted to get really lean, your body, if anything, is actually a bit more primed for fat storage. Also;

2) that this relationship is based on observations of individuals who aren't resistance training. If you start lifting weights this drastically changes the game.

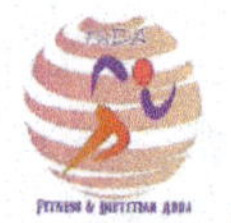

112

Nutrient partitioning in your now highly active skeletal muscle is much more favorable for muscle gain as you are providing a stimulus for growth and regularly depleting your muscle of energy and pushing them to become energy efficient and adapt. If it was true that individuals with a high body fat couldn't gain muscle mass effectively, sumo wrestlers wouldn't have the highest recorded lean body masses of any athlete...but they do. Likewise, super heavyweight powerlifters would be weaker

than weight classes below them, but they aren't.

Now don't get me wrong, this isn't a license to go on a dreamer permabulk! But rather, I'm saying don't be the guy who is afraid to enter a surplus because they aren't 8% body fat, or the gal who is afraid because they aren't 16%.

There probably should be some limit to how high your body fat is before you decide it would be better to cut versus bulk, but it's for logistical reasons not "anabolic resistance". Essentially, you don't want to only get a month or two out of your gaining phase before you have to diet.

If you are a powerlifter you don't want to be too far above your weight class, and for bodybuilders, you don't want to be too far off stage weight. In either case, the inevitable diet to come will be unnecessarily hard or long if you are. Likewise, for recreational lifters, you probably don't want to be so high in body fat at the start of a gaining phase that you aren't happy with your body shortly after starting it. Essentially, in each case you want enough of a runway to be able to spend at least a few months in a surplus.

My rough guidelines are a maximum of ~15% body fat for men and ~23% body fat for women for beginning a gaining phase. After starting, allow your body fat to climb ~3–5% in the course of a gaining phase before you do a brief 'mini cut' to clean things up a tad before you rinse and repeat. A general recommendation (for those who aren't starting with a high body fat level) is to have a minimum of a 4:1 ratio of the time spent in a gaining phase vs a cutting phase. Thus, if you spent four months in a surplus putting on muscle, you earned yourself no more than one month to do a mini cut.

Now, the tough part is actually assessing your body fat level. Everyone stores body fat differently. Also, having more or less muscle mass can make a given body fat level look better or worse. So in the end, just make your best guess as to whether you are below or above the cut-off. If you are somewhere in the range where either a cutting or gaining phase could be appropriate and you can't tell where you fall and what you should do, don't worry, it doesn't matter which you choose to do. You hopefully realized that though, now that you are no longer under the false impression that your gaining phase will be sabotaged if you don't start it lean enough.

About Cardio Use for Fat Loss

Also, the caloric deficit doesn't have to come entirely from the diet, and you probably guessed that adding some cardiovascular work to expend more energy rather than restricting your energy intake alone could also be useful.

A simple way to estimate energy expenditure during cardio requires you to determine a **Rating of Perceived Exertion (RPE)** during exercise.

This can be simply done by considering how hard it feels on a scale from 1 to 10. If you also track the time spent performing the cardio, and if you know your body weight, you can estimate caloric expenditure with reasonable accuracy. You burn approximately ~0.2, ~0.45 and ~0.7 kcal per 10 minutes per pound of body weight doing light (RPE 2 to 4 out of 10), moderate (RPE 5 to 7 out of 10) and vigorous (RPE 8 to 10 out of 10) cardio respectively, above what you would normally be burning doing everyday light activity in that same time period.

DEFICIENCY DISEASES

A person may be getting enough food to eat, but sometimes the food may not contain a particular nutrient. If this continues over a long period of time, the person may suffer from its deficiency.

Deficiency of one or more nutrients can cause diseases or disorders in our body. Diseases that occur due to lack of nutrients over a long period are called deficiency diseases. If a person does not get enough proteins in his/her food for a long time, he/she is likely to have stunted growth, swelling of face, discoloration of hair, skin diseases and diarrhoea. If the diet is deficient in both carbohydrates and proteins for a long period of time, the growth may stop completely. Such a person becomes very lean and thin and so weak that he/she may not even be able to move. Deficiency of different vitamins and minerals may also result in certain diseases or disorders.

All deficiency diseases can be prevented by taking a balanced diet.

_______________By_Mr._Hitesh_Andel_______________

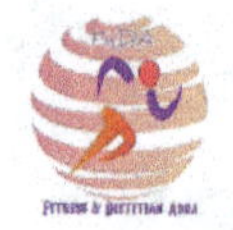

114

Chapter 11: Ketogenic Diet

OVERVIEW

This has been a real hype in recent years. It has been treated as a God-sent magical diet. While it works great, trust me, it's no more superior to any other structured diet, considering only fat loss as the result, if you keep the basic variables the same, that is, your intake and your expenditure in terms of energy, your total protein intake and your training.

A keto diet is well known for being a low carb diet, where the body produces ketones in the liver to be used as energy. It's referred to by many different names – ketogenic diet, low carb diet, low carb high fat, etc. When you eat something high in carbs, your body will produce glucose and insulin.

Glucose is the easiest molecule for your body to convert and use as energy, so it will be chosen over any other energy source.

By lowering the intake of carbs, the body is induced into a state known as ketosis. Ketosis is a natural process the body initiates to help us survive when food intake is low. During this state, we produce ketones, which are produced from the breakdown of fats in the liver. The end goal of a properly maintained keto diet is to force your body into this metabolic state. We don't do this through starvation of calories, but through starvation of carbohydrates.

Ketogenic diet or keto is basically a diet where you will have absolutely minimum carbs say 20-30gms max. This will force the body to utilize fat as a primary source of fuel thereby aiding fat loss.

Our bodies are extremely adaptive to what you put into it – when you overload it with fats and take away carbohydrates, it will begin to burn ketones as the main energy source.

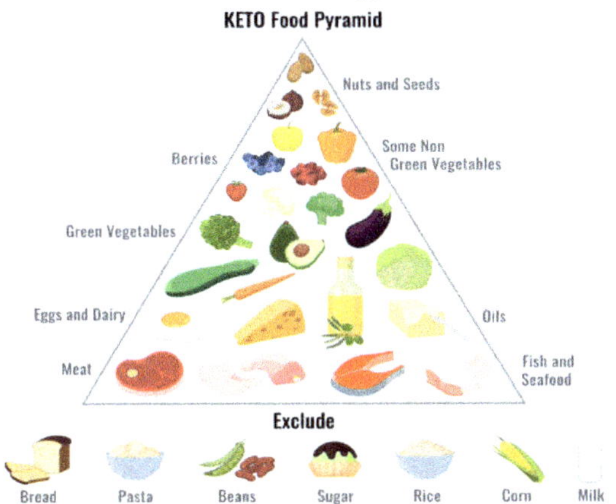

For **Atkins**, I suggest you use the 5:35:60 macro ratio i.e. 5 portions of Carbs, 35 portions of Protein and 60 portions of Fat.
Now for example,
My BMR is around 1500 and my TDEE (total daily energy expenditure is 2000) so my macro breakdown for Keto will be:
25gms of Carbs, 200gms of Protein, and 133gms of Fat.
Now we will build a sample diet around this. Like I've mentioned earlier, I like to keep things simple and hence I use food that I use daily and is easily available.

For Atkins, following are the BEST CHOICES for me
- Paneer (per100gm–Fat 20 gm, Protein ~ 20 gm, Carb1.5 gm)
- Amul cheese (1 slice–Fat 5 gm, ~Protein 4 gm, Carbs–negligible)
- Extra Virgin Coconut Oil (per100gm--Fat 86gm)
- Flaxseed (per 100gm – Fat 42gm, ~Protein 18gm, Carbs 29gm)
- Spinach (or any other dark green vegetables for fiber)

FOOD
AROUND 8AM
Breakfast 50gm Paneer 1 Cheese Slice
4 Egg Whites

AROUND 11AM
50gm Paneer 1 Cheese Slice

1PM LUNCH
100gm Paneer
1 Bowl of Spinach or any of your favorite vegetable,

Snacks
Paneer Cubes sauteed in Extra Virgin Coconut Oil

9PM DINNER
100gm Paneer
1 Bowl of Spinach or any of your favorite vegetable

NOTE:
1. Paneer (per100gm fat20gm,protein~20gm, carb 1.5gm).
2. Amul Cheese (1 Slice–Fat 5gm, ~Protein 4gm, Carbs-negligible)
3. Spinach (or any other dark green vegetables for fibre)
4. Extra virgin coconut oil (per100gm--fat86gm)

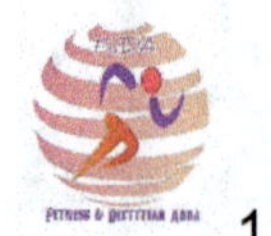

This was just an approximated version and the diet will vary for every individual. Let me remind you again that this information is to help you understand how to make a customized diet plan and not to give you a readymade plan.

Ketosis within your body will start typically 2-3 days after you start this diet and you will start seeing quick results soon. You may get a urine test done to see if your body is producing more ketones than usual, or you can simply test it with urine analysis sticks.

Also if you lose 1-2 kgs in the initial 2-3 days, don't start jumping! Like I mentioned, it would be your water weight associated with the glycogen that will be depleted. Although, you can lose up to 4-5 kgs in 4 weeks of this diet (varies for every individual again).

Please note - A lot of people recommend a diet to be done every week. However, from my experience, I have noticed that the body gets smooth and retains a lot of water. It is a good idea to stay on keto for at least 4 weeks continuously before having carbs again in a refeed.

Also sometimes, people start consuming more protein thinking it will help. However, it doesn't really help that way since you may get thrown out of ketosis with higher intake of protein too. It would be wise to have a higher protein intake in the initial weeks until the body gets keto adapted. *Once ketosis is achieved, the protein intake can be reduced to around 15-20% of the diet.*

Ketogenic Nutrition :

What you eat really depends how fast you want to get into a ketogenic state. The more restrictive you are on your carbohydrates (less than 15g per day), the faster you will enter ketosis.

Normally, anywhere between 20-30g of net carbs is recommended for every day dieting – but the lower you keep your glucose levels, the better the overall results will be.

You might be asking, "What's a net carb?" It's simple really! *The net carbs are your total dietary carbohydrates, minus the total fiber.*

Let's say for example you want to eat some broccoli (1 cup) –

- There are a total of 6g carbohydrates in 1 cup.
- There is also 2g of fiber in 1 cup.
- So, we take the 6g (total carbs) and subtract the 2g (dietary fiber). This will give us our net carbs of 4g.

KETO MACROS

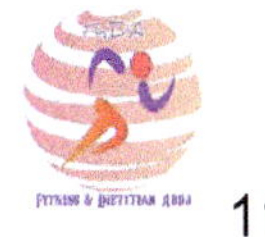

Your nutrient intake should be something around **70% fats, 25% protein, and 5% carbohydrate**. You want to keep your carbohydrates limited, coming mostly from vegetables, nuts, and dairy. Don't eat any refined carbohydrates such as wheat (breads, pastas, cereals, roti), starch (potatoes, beans, channe, Lentils,) or fruit.

Dark green and leafy is always the best choice. Most of your meals should be protein with vegetables, and an extra side of fat. Chicken breast, paneer, fish, tofu with vegetables would be awesome.

If you're finding yourself hungry throughout the day, you can snack on nuts, seeds, or peanut butter to curb your appetite.

Benefits of a Keto Diet

- **Cholesterol**. A keto diet has shown to improve triglyceride levels and cholesterol levels most associated with arterial buildup.
- **Weight Loss**. As your body is burning fat as the main source of energy, you will essentially be using your fat stores as an energy source while in a fasting state.
- **Blood Sugar**. The decrease of LDL cholesterol over time and have shown to eliminate ailments such as type 2 diabetes.
- **Energy**. By giving your body a better and more reliable energy source, you will feel more energized during the day. Fats are shown to be the most effective molecule to burn as fuel.
- **Hunger**. Fat is naturally more satisfying and ends up leaving us in a satiated ("full") state.

Cyclic Ketogenic Diet (CKD) AND CHEAT MEALS

Cheat Meal is that meal in your diet where you can have any food that you like and it can be absolutely anything from a full-fledged ice cream sundae to your favorite biryani. Anyone with a *body fat percentage below 10%* can have a cheat meal after an induction period of approximately 4 weeks of following a ketogenic diet strictly. This is done to boost your *leptin* levels, which is one of the most critical hormones for losing fat.

If you are getting results and your weight loss has not stalled, then there is no need for a cheat meal and you can just keep playing with your calories. Just don't bring it down to the levels you started with.

The Cyclic Ketogenic Diet, also popularly known as CKD should be followed by people who have **body fat levels below 8%**.

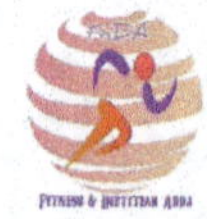

118

People up to 10% can also follow it but they should have a decent amount of muscle mass. The main principle behind a cyclic ketogenic diet is the depletion and super compensation of your glycogen stores like I explained earlier. It is very critical for your sarcoplasmic growth. Now, even CKD can be done only once you are keto induced. So it is advised to follow a strict ketogenic diet for a period of at least 3-4 weeks. This induction phase is very important and further determines the success of your CKD. Some people tend to jump directly on CKD without getting properly induced, which is nothing short of a disaster.

So here is the correct method of doing CKD:
You have to get keto induced for a period of 3-4 weeks (make sure you're around 8% BF), then you move to CKD. You stay on Keto for a period of 5-6 days (depending on your goal), and then load carbs for a period of 24-48 hours depending on your muscle mass, sensitivity towards carbs and a lot of other factors.

A typical CKD cycle for a week would look like this:
MONDAY	- keto
TUESDAY	- keto
WEDNESDAY	- keto
THURSDAY	- keto
FRIDAY	- keto

SATURDAY morning, you need to do a depletion workout (high intensity, full body, high volume, high rep workout done to make sure your glycogen levels are completely depleted) after which you will start taking a combination of glucose + protein, every 2 hours for the next 8 hours along with some simple carbs. In the subsequent 16 hours, you can eat solid meals like rice, chicken, pasta, oats and anything else you want. The amount of carbs that you need to take, depends on
your lean body weight. The typical formula is to have around 6-8 gm per kg of your lean body weight, so for a 70kg guy with 10% bf, that would come at around 500-600gms of carbs. However, this formula is highly flawed and can often lead to excess carbs. Instead, I'd suggest eating 50gm carbs every 2 hours in the next 16 hours and see how your body reacts.

On SUNDAY morning, you should look fuller, more defined and more muscular. If you are holding water, or you are looking flat, it means, either the carbs were too less or they were too many. So it takes a little trial and error to hit the right amount. Again, this you will have to figure out on your own with some practice and see what works for

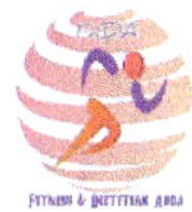

you. On Sunday you can either continue to load carbs, or if you have had too many on Saturday and are holding water, then do some cardio to burn off the excess calories and you can switch to keto or eat carbs at your maintenance calories. Some people make use of the period and do cheats as well, which is fine

since everything you eat is primarily used by your body to fill up your depleted glycogen stores. So sweets, ice-creams, candies, cookies, biryani etc. are all allowed, however make sure your total fat intake on these 1-2 days is less than 15% of your maintenance calories.

Also, make sure you do your depletion workout with maximum intensity, as the only way to super compensate your glycogen levels is by making sure it is completely depleted in the first place.

What happens when we stop taking Carbohydrates in our Diet:

When you don't get enough carbohydrates, the level of sugar in your blood may drop to below the normal range (70-99 mg/dL), causing hypoglycemia. Your body then starts to burn fat for energy, leading to ketosis.

In the process of breaking down fat, the body produces ketones, which are then removed by the body through frequent and increased urination. This may lead to dehydration and flu-like symptoms, such as fatigue, **dizziness, irritability, nausea, and muscle soreness**.

"*Ketosis* is a process that happens when your body doesn't have enough carbohydrates to burn for energy. Instead, it burns fat and makes things called ketones, which it can use for fuel."

Symptoms of hypoglycemia include:

- Hunger
- Shakiness
- Dizziness
- Confusion
- Difficulty speaking
- Feeling anxious or weak

Symptoms of ketosis include:

- Mental fatigue
- Bad breath
- Nausea and headache
- Painful swelling of the joints and kidney stones in severe ketosis.

_______________________By_Mr._Hitesh_Andel_______________________

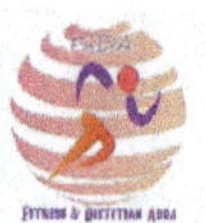

120

Chapter 12: Supplementation

Supplement

A dietary supplement is a manufactured product intended to supplement one's diet by taking a pill, capsule, tablet, powder, or liquid. A supplement can provide nutrients either extracted from food sources or that are synthetic in order to increase the quantity of their consumption.

There are infinite numbers of supplements available in the market these days, if you start buying them all, you'll probably have no money left in your pocket. See these products work, they have years of solid research backing up their claims, but there are two things to consider :

1. It's just 5% of your entire 100% and

2. For this mere 5%, it costs a BOMB!

Who has the money for this idiotic advantage of 5%, right? Instead give 100% in your diet and training efforts. Here, I'll only cover the most basic and most essential supplements.

Protein

You need this no matter how good your diet is, don't fall for expensive isolates though, blends are good too. How much? 1-1.8 gm per kg of lean body weight is decent.

Protein powder is a popular nutritional supplement. Protein is an essential macronutrient that helps build muscle, repair tissue, and make enzymes and hormones. Using protein powder may also aid weight loss and help people tone their muscles.

Whey Protein

Whey protein has one of the best quality amino acid profiles and has been shown to stimulate muscle protein synthesis to greater degrees compared to other forms. Whey protein is acid soluble and thus is digested quickly which increases amino acid delivery into the blood.

Casein Protein

Casein Protein is another milk derivative protein similar to whey. The main difference between whey and casein is the slower digestion rates. Casein does not stimulate muscle protein synthesis to the same degree as whey.

Egg Protein

Egg protein is another great alternative for those who may have milk allergies or who are unable to properly digest whey or casein.

Eggs are also a high-quality protein with adequate levels of leucine and other essential amino acids. In fact, egg protein is second to whey protein in leucine content. Until recently, eggs were the gold standard protein source and actually used as the reference for measuring protein quality because of their high EAA profile and digestibility rates. For whole eggs, not only are they one of the best protein sources on the planet, but they also provide a ton of nutrients, making them one of the healthiest whole foods in the world.

Soy Protein

Soy protein has less leucine compared to whey which is the key amino acid to signal our body to lay down new muscle tissue.

Plant Protein

All animal proteins are complete, meaning that they contain all of the essential amino acids required for muscle growth and repair. Sadly, plant-based proteins are not, but by combining certain plant-based proteins with enzymes you can speed up digestion and cause a significantly larger spike in muscle protein synthesis.

Creatine

It gives you more energy to lift! Literally! When lifting heavy weights, your body primarily uses ATP and CP (Creatine phosphate) stores, however these are very limited and you cannot push any further until the body makes more ATP from glycogen again. Also most of this ATP actually exists in the body in the form of ADP (adenosine di-phosphate).

When Creatine monohydrate is introduced in the body, it binds to the phosphorus inside the body and exists as Creatine phosphate. Now this Creatine phosphate during heavy workouts gives its phosphate to ADP to form ATP, this happens much faster than glycogen to ATP conversion thereby there's a notable increase in your strength.

Creatine is one of the most well researched supplements available in the market and should be used by anyone who lifts weight.

Now there's a common myth among the bodybuilding community, that Creatine retains water. So let's address that. First of all, what do you mean by water retention? The water is stored in your muscle cells as well as outside of your muscle cells under the skin.

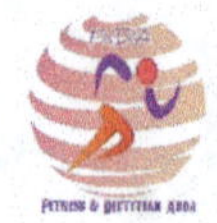

This extracellular water stored under the skin is called Water Retention. It's a defense mechanism employed by the body to keep you hydrated all the time.

Now Creatine draws water directly into the muscles and not into the extracellular skin, which is a good thing. Tell this to the experts and they'll be rolling their eyes now. Most of the time, these people stop drinking water all together and stop consuming sodium as well.

Now sodium is one major electrolyte that helps in regulation of water in the body. So when the body detects low levels of sodium and water, the hormone aldosterone is triggered, which further as a part of the body's defense mechanism tries to hang onto the water, thereby causing water retention intracellular as well as extracellular. And people thought it was due to Creatine.

BCAA

You don't really need it if you have enough protein intake which has a complete amino acid profile. BCAA or branched chain amino acids are basically essential amino acids which are synthesized in the body, namely *leucine, isoleucine and valine* along with many other amino acids.

However, what makes these BCAA's more important is the role they play. These amino acids are being used by the body for energy when you're lifting heavy weights. And if the body starts making these amino acids it will not manufacture other amino acids at the same speed. And we know that all the amino acids are required for building proteins which are nothing but chains of amino acids.

So it is always a good idea to supplement these essential amino acids, thereby giving the body enough time to make all other amino acids, further leading to more muscle protein synthesis.

However, if your protein intake for the day is sufficient, then you do not need to supplement with BCAA.

ZMA

ZMA or *Zinc Magnesium Aspartate* is a mineral supplement that is a combination of Zinc Monomethionine Aspartate, Magnesium Aspartate and Vitamin B6. The reason ZMA has become popular amongst athletes and people who do resistance training is because it supplements mainly with zinc and magnesium which is studied to be deficient in people who train.

Zinc has been proven to be vital for the activity of more than 300 enzymes. Zinc contains enzymes aid in macronutrient

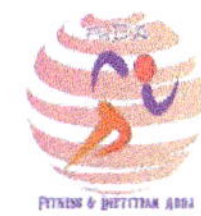

123

metabolism and cell replication, which as we know are key biochemical functions that correspond to recovery and growth.

Zinc has shown to have positive effects on anabolic hormone profile, particularly testosterone. It increases free serum testosterone levels which is particularly important in older men as their testosterone levels start to decline with age.

Why supplement with ZMA?

It is not really necessary if you have ample intake of these minerals from your diet. But if not, you might want to consider its use. Lower levels of zinc and magnesium are either due to sweating while training where you lose a lot of minerals and electrolytes or due to poor diet.

ZMA improves sleep- studies show that people suffering from mild to moderate Insomnia seem to improve with oral magnesium therapy. Long term sleep deprivation causes magnesium deficiency and improving the magnesium intake can help with sleep. ZMA improves REM (rapid eye movement) cycles of sleep. The better your sleep, the more you recover and assimilate nutrients. The list goes on; I'd suggest sticking with the basics.

Micronutrients

Your Multivitamin/multimineral tabs. They come cheap, and it's a good idea to take them. You may not realize this but if your diet doesn't have chromium in it, you will suffer poor metabolism.

Let me explain, even though chromium is required in micrograms, it is an essential cofactor for proper functioning of your hormone insulin. And you know how important insulin is. This is just one example showing how important these micronutrients in your body can be. There are a total of more than 26 such vitamins and minerals that are required for optimum health by your body every day. Unfortunately, there is no single food that will provide you the full spectrum, hence supplementation becomes all the more essential. Multivitamins and minerals tabs can do that for you.

Having a balanced diet can take care of most of the micronutrients, however supplementation of the following is always beneficial and is even recommended:

Vitamin C, and for vegetarians - Vitamin–B (thiamin, riboflavin, niacin, and so on).

Don't forget fish oil capsules or flaxseed oil for omega-3 and omega-6 fatty acids. Remember they are required by your brain. Similarly, garlic is a very beneficial herb.

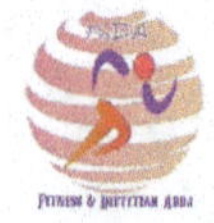

124

(I'll Discuss the Indian Spices or Herbs in Next Chapter) Try to explore more herbs and check out their benefits. A fish oil capsule will cost you more but flax seed you can get for 140rs/kg in the market.

HORMONES

I won't be going deep into the endocrine system, but it will be helpful to you to get the basics of a few important hormones right.

So what are hormones?

Hormones are special chemical messengers that pass messages between different parts of your body and control various important functions in your body. They coordinate complex processes like growth, fertility and metabolism.

You have facial hair? Hormones.

You have good muscles naturally? Hormones.

You feel very energetic? Hormones.

Your menstruation to your thyroid functions – Hormones.

You are diabetic? Well, hormones.

Hormones play a very important role in everything that your body goes through. Let's look at a few important hormones.

Insulin-

Insulin has always been propagated as the muscle building hormone and even as the fat storing hormone. Truth is, it does both and you don't need to fret much about it. It's a hormone that helps you stay stable, by keeping your blood glucose levels stable when it tends to rise due to incoming carb intake. It "opens up" the cells to take the incoming glucose in.

Insulin is a hormone made by the pancreas that allows your body to use sugar (glucose) from carbohydrates in the food that you eat for energy or to store glucose for future use. Insulin helps keep your blood sugar level from getting too high (hyperglycemia) or too low (hypoglycemia).

The cells in your body need sugar for energy. However, sugar cannot go into most of your cells directly. After you eat food and your blood sugar level rises, cells in your pancreas (known as beta cells) are signalled to release insulin into your bloodstream. Insulin then attaches to and signals cells to absorb sugar from the bloodstream. Insulin is often described as a "key," which unlocks the cell to allow sugar to enter the cell and be used for energy.

Glucagon-

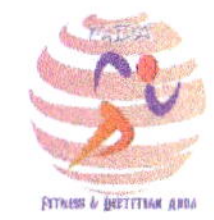

We discussed how insulin helps keep the blood glucose level stable by helping the body take in the excess glucose. Glucagon does the exact opposite by helping the blood glucose remain stable by bringing in supply of glucose when blood glucose is low, by breaking down the stored glycogen in the liver.

So insulin and glucagon are interlinked, and it's no surprise that both of them are produced in the pancreas itself.

Testosterone-

Now testosterone is the primary male hormone which gives men their "male" characteristic, from voice to facial hair. It helps maintain proper health in men and also helps to build muscles. Now testosterone is a male hormone, but it doesn't mean that women don't produce it. Even women produce it, but much less than men. Women are more sensitive to this hormone. A healthy testosterone level is important for you for proper muscle gain and fat loss. So make sure your micronutrients are on point and that you are not on a hypocaloric diet for a long time. (Note – there is a difference between calorie deficit and hypocaloric. Hypocaloric diet here means severe deficit for a long time.)

The Best testosterone booster in nature is lifting heavy weights. If you lift weights, your testosterone production gets better, thereby aiding in muscle build up and strength gains (in women, "toning" is essentially muscle build up itself, along with fat loss. Lifting weights will help you do that instead of aerobics)

Estrogen-

Estrogen is the female counterpart of testosterone. It makes a woman, a woman. It is responsible for the development and regulation of the female reproductive system and secondary sex charateristics. Now there are several different types of estrogen too, but that is beyond the scope of this book for now. One thing to remember here is, it is a very important hormone for women. And lifting weights will NOT bring it down to affect your health.

Another concern among men is about the increase of estrogen in their bodies due to soya consumption. That won't happen unless you eat 1 kilo raw soya everyday continuously for months at a stretch. So there's nothing to worry about.

Leptin-

Leptin is a very important hormone in your body that's essential for fat loss. It is like your fuel indicator that signals your brain about the

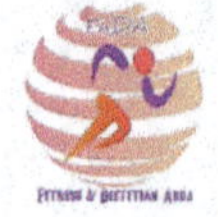

126

availability of food, and based on that your brain holds on to your body's fat stores or goes easy on them to release them for use. That's directly related to metabolic adaptation. This hormone goes down when you are on a caloric deficit for too long, and the effect is more if carbs are omitted from the diet. This is the reason why a refeed helps. A well-timed and well-placed refeed can help you lose more by raising your leptin levels after a short dieting phase.

Ghrelin-

This hormone is also known as the hunger hormone. It signals your body to feed it more. This hormone goes up when you are on a caloric deficit for long and are dieting up. That's why you feel hungry. So the next time you feel hungry, don't think that your body lacks energy or energy stores. It has a lot of fat stores that it can use. It's just the ghrelin in action.

Cortisol-

In the fitness community, cortisol is seen as the *villain*. Truth is, it is neutral. Depends on how it functions and the scenario it functions in. It is a catabolic hormone that helps in the metabolism of fat, protein and carbohydrate – all three. So even your fat loss is dependent on cortisol. However, excess amounts of cortisol for extended time periods is bad as it can metabolise your muscle mass too. Cortisol is released in response to stress and low blood glucose concentration.
TIP – Minimize your stress, be on a good diet and make sure you take your micronutrients. Get involved in activities that you like doing. Pursue a hobby, meditate. It will not just help you with your cortisol but also lead a good life. My belief is health, not only in your body but also in your mind.

_____________________By_Mr._Hitesh_Andel_____________________

Chapter 13: Indian Spices

Introduction

Spices are natural plant or vegetable products or a mixture of both like a dried seed, fruit, root or bark which can be either in whole or ground form which possess preservative, colourant, antioxidant, antibiotic and antiseptic properties. They supply calcium, Vitamin B, Vitamin C, iron, carotene and other oxidants. They also have very low fat content. They are also useful in fighting germs, intensifying salivary flow, checking infection, cleanse the oral cavity and protect the mucous membrane. They act as stimuli to the digestive system.

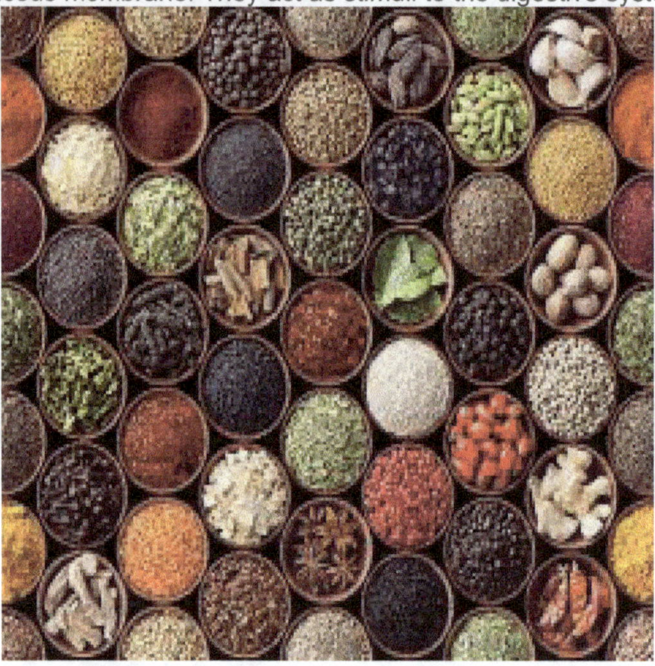

Origin of Spice in India

Indian spices have a history which is more than 7000 years old. It has always been a leading spice consuming, producing and exporting country of the world and spices play a leading role in India's national economy.

Health Benefits Of Spices

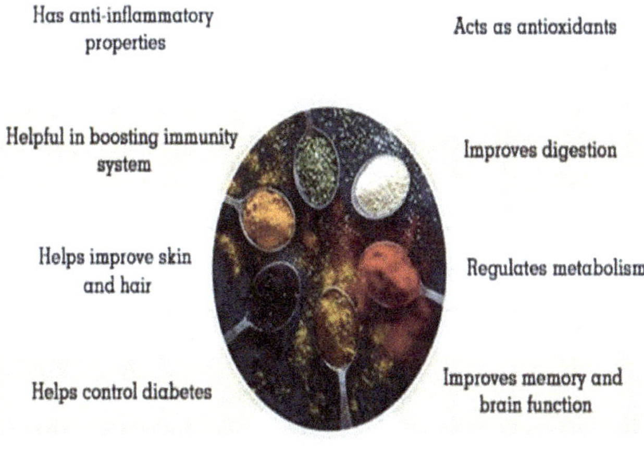

Divisions of Spices
Spices are broadly divided into two main divisions-
Major spices and Minor Spices.
Major categories are Ginger, turmeric, pepper, cardamom, chillies etc.
Minor categories are aniseed, ajwain, celery, cumin, coriander, fennel, onion, garlic, fenugreek, saffron, vanilla etc.

Ayurveda and Spices
Ayurveda is a form of alternative medicine which is natural and holistic and is native to India. Many spices are made use of in their medicines as they have no side effects and are very useful in the treatment of the diseases.

Spices
It is difficult to name all the spices, but I'm trying to mention some of the well known Indian Spices and their Health Benefits.

Kerala is the major state leading in pepper production in India. India is the foremost exporter and producer of chillies.

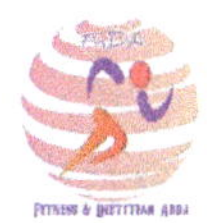

129

Uses and Benefits of Spices

1. **Asafoetida (Hing)**- Used for seasoning food and helps to relieve stomach ache caused by gas and in whooping cough.
2. **Bay Leaf (Tej Patta)**- It is used to add special flavour to the food and its oil has antifungal and antibacterial properties.
3. **Cardamom (Elaichi)**- It is used to give flavour and smell in cooking particularly in sweet dishes and also in the pharmaceutical sector. It helps in digestive disorders and controlling bad breath.
4. **Chilli (Lal mirch)**- It is used for adding hot flavour to food. The antioxidants in the chilli help to contain cholesterol and help in burning calories.
5. **Cinnamon (Dalchini)**- It is used for preparing masalas and for seasoning food. It reduces blood cholesterol and helps in the production of insulin.
6. **Clove(Laung)**- It is used in seasoning and preparing masalas. It helps in sore gums and tooth ache and during chest pain, cough, cold, fever and digestive problems.
7. **Coriander (Dhania)**- The leaves as well as seeds are used in cooking. It helps in coping with allergies, sore throat, hay fever, digestive problems and can be used externally for rheumatism and aching joints.
8. **Cumin(Jeera)**- It is used in cooking and is a good source of iron and keeps one immune from diseases. Cumin seeds boiled in water helps in coping with dysentery.
9. **Curry leaves (Karipatha)**- It is used in cooking and for seasoning food. They are used in herbal medicines and for reducing blood sugar.
10. **Fennel (Saunf)**- It is used in cooking and helps in digestion after eating, relieves nausea, gas, indigestion, bloating etc.
11. **Fenugreek (Methi)**- The leaves are used as a vegetable and the seeds are used in cooking. It helps in lowering cholesterol and blood sugar and tea made from it increases breast milk.
12. **Garlic(Lassan)**- It is used in cooking and helps to cope with cough and cold and has antibiotic properties.
13. **Ginger (Adrak)**- It is used in cooking and helps in cough and cold and helps to avoid digestive problems.
14. **Mustard(Rai)**- It is used in cooking and its oil also is used in many countries. It consists of Omega 3 fatty acids and is an excellent source of zinc, manganese, calcium, iron, proteins etc. It helps in good skin, hair and is used in body massage.

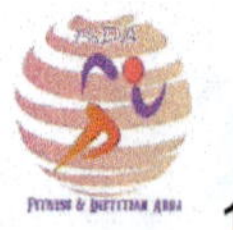

130

15. **Nutmeg (Jaiphal)**- It is used in cooking for garnishing and preparing masalas. It is also used in perfumes, shampoos and soaps. It helps in treating bad breath, heart disorders and asthma.
16. **Black Pepper (Kaali Mirch)**- It is used in cooking and garnishing. It helps in coping with muscle pains, cold, cough, infections and digestive problems.
17. **Saffron (Kesar or Zaffran)**- It is used in cooking and flavouring as well as beauty products. It helps in relieving cough, cold, asthma and coping with skin diseases.
18. **Star Anise (Chakra Phool)**- It is used in cooking. It helps in digestion, avoiding bad breath and its oil is useful for rheumatism.
19. **Turmeric (Haldi)**- It is used in cooking and in skin care products. It helps in healing cuts and wounds and in skin problems. It also helps in coping with diabetes.

_______________________By_Mr._Hitesh_Andel_______________

Bibliography _:_
https://www.wikipedia.com
https://www.fittr.com/
https://www.health.india.com
https://www.indianfood.indiannetzone.com
https://www.myfitnesspal.com
https://www.healthifyme.com
Self test and client results.